"This book helps you to obtain the quality of care that your clinicians want to provide—and that you have every right to receive."

—Laura Weil, Director Emeritus, Master's Program in Health Advocacy, Sarah Lawrence College

"Elizabeth Bailey's book puts a human face on the devastating toll medical errors have on patients and their families and clearly shows that when we use checklists to improve the quality of care, we save lives. I have seen the power of this important tool; using checklists in a hospital setting, we nearly eliminated bloodstream infections, a preventable disease that kills about as many people every year as breast cancer. Imagine what the simple checklists in this book can do for you."

—Peter J. Pronovost, MD, PhD, FCCM, coauthor, with Eric Vohr, of *Safe Patients, Smart Hospitals: How One Doctor's Checklist Can Help Us Change Health Care from the Inside Out*

"Elizabeth Bailey learned what could go wrong in a hospital the hard way: by watching her elderly father endure a long in-patient nightmare. Six years later, she has turned that system into a book."
—*USA Today*

"*The Patient's Checklist* should be in the hands of all families in the event of a hospital stay. The information could save your or a loved one's life."

—Christiane Northrup, MD, author of the *New York Times* best sellers *Women's Bodies, Women's Wisdom* and *The Wisdom of Menopause*

The Patient's Checklist

The Patient's Checklist

10 Simple Hospital Checklists to Keep You Safe, Sane, and Organized

Elizabeth Bailey

New York

Copyright © 2011, 2020 by Elizabeth Bailey

Previously published by Sterling Publishing

Cover design by LeeAnn Falciani

Cover copyright © 2020 by Hachette Book Group, Inc.

Hachette Go, an imprint of Hachette Books
Hachette Book Group
1290 Avenue of the Americas
New York, NY 10104
HachetteGo.com
Facebook.com/HachetteGo
Instagram.com/HachetteGo

Previously published by Sterling: 2012

First Hachette Go Paperback Edition: September 2020

First eBook Edition: June 2020

Hachette Books is a division of Hachette Book Group, Inc.

The Hachette Go and Hachette Books names and logos are trademarks of Hachette Book Group, Inc.

The publisher is not responsible for websites (or their content) that are not owned by the publisher.

Library of Congress Cataloging-in-Publication Data has been applied for.

Library of Congress Control Number: 2020938925

ISBNs: 978-0-306-92465-1 (paperback); 978-0-306-92466-8 (ebook)

Printed in the United States of America

LSC-C

10 9 8 7 6 5 4 3 2 1

Illness is the night-side of life, a more onerous citizenship. Everyone who is born holds dual citizenship, in the kingdom of the well and the kingdom of the sick. Although we all prefer to use only the good passport, sooner or later each of us is obliged, at least for a spell, to identify ourselves as citizens of the other place.

—Susan Sontag, *Illness as Metaphor*

Contents

Prologue: How I Came to Write This Book   xi

Introduction   1

How to Use the Checklists   7

THE CHECKLISTS

1 Before You Go   11

2 What to Bring   27

3 During Your Stay   35

4 Master Medication List   45

5 Daily Medication Log   61

6 Daily Journal   77

7 Discharge Plan   101

8 Insurance   113

9 Doctor Contacts   123

10 Family & Friends Contacts   135

Resources   145

Introduction Statistics Sources   151

Index   153

About the Author   161

Prologue

HOW I CAME TO WRITE THIS BOOK

The more serious the illness, the more important it is for you to fight back, mobilizing all your resources—spiritual, emotional, intellectual, physical.

—Norman Cousins, *Anatomy of an Illness*

Ten years ago when I began to write the first edition of *The Patient's Checklist* I was looking for the soul in high-tech medicine. Today, on the eve of the publication of this revised second edition, the whole world is engulfed by COVID-19—a virus that remains a scientific mystery as it mercilessly causes untold human suffering and death and wreaks economic havoc everywhere.

Hospitals and the delivery of care in our country are in the news 24/7. What is going on in public health has asked us all to think about our personal health. All of us can see two things clearly about the state of our hospitals. We clap nightly for our heroic frontline staff who put their lives at risk every moment of every day to save us. At the same time, the scales have dropped from our collective eyes as we see the catastrophic systemic problems with our market-driven for-profit health-care delivery system—not having enough personal protective equipment (PPE), inadequate testing and contact tracing, dwindling reserves of a whole range of critical equipment and medicine, and the gross inequity of access to care. It's all about cost not care.

What we are witnessing in real time is a deeply flawed, unfair, complex health-care delivery system that has ignored that, at its core, the art of medicine remains the human-to-human connection between patient and provider essential to healing illness or injury. More than ever we recognize this is the soul of medicine, even as masks and gowns and quarantine present physical obstacles.

The initial impetus for this book was my rage and grief about what happened to my Dad, a story I tell below. I blamed the doctors and nurses—to me the human face of a gawping profit machine called the U.S. health-care system. To fight back I went to graduate school for health advocacy and wound up working in a renowned hospital as an inpatient advocate.

Very quickly I was disabused of my "hospital staff = uncaring clinicians" mindset. Working as a hospital patient advocate opened my eyes to the crushing demands that our for-profit health-care system places on frontline staff. Of course, there were some doctors or nurses who seemed less than empathetic or impatient—but I wondered how much of this was due to the way hospitals actually work. Everything was a money squeeze to cut costs and boost profits—understaffing, scarcity of supplies, and the relentless grind of punching in billing codes to a patient's electronic medical record—as opposed to the creation of a useful, open-notes document describing a patient's actual health status. All of this creates countless opportunities for error to occur.

Patient-centered care has been the buzzword for the past decade. Conferences meet. Experts write books. We all intrinsically understand that a collaborative approach involving physicians, nurses, patients, and families makes for better, safer care. The slogan for Patient Safety Week is "Be aware for safe care." *The Patient's Checklist* was premised on creating a tool kit for patients and families to feel empowered and effectively play their parts in complex hospital care because each patient must be seen as a whole person. The user-friendly checklists trust that with a little bit of help patients and families can be effective in monitoring daily care. The stats that introduce each checklist are not meant to terrify but to alert those entering the hospital that errors are real and vigilance is essential. The real patient stories captured in "hospital spotlights" are lessons learned the hard way—my hope is that by sharing them, others can avoid the experience. The fundamental takeaway I hope is to prevent the communication failures that are the root cause of most medical errors.

COVID-19 threatens to make irrelevant all we know about best practices for hospital care premised on involving patients and their families to improve safety and outcomes because it demands isolation in an acute care setting by separating loved ones and caregivers at this critical time. All patients, COVID-19 or otherwise, enter the hospital alone; family members cannot be at their bedside. Though we are finding work-arounds to connect families with patients remotely because their input is essential, it is still a work in progress. The pandemic has made it clear that families not only are the chief guardians of patient safety but also have always been the main providers of essential comfort care, the high-touch in high-tech medicine. Both of these critical components to safe, optimal care are absent when patients must be alone in the hospital.

Who knows what recovery will look like—for patients, providers, and hospitals—once this pandemic has been vanquished? I suspect we will see new behavioral norms—like frequent handwashing—that will have profound impacts on patient safety by dramatically reducing hospital infection rates. A simple act. I suspect we will see more clearly the necessity of bedside comfort care—of holding a hand, of being present—because it was at risk of being swept aside by COVID-19. More than ever, we will see the absolute necessity of collaboration among patients, families, and health-care providers for the best outcomes.

At eighty-one, my father was still practicing law, exercising daily, and living independently in New York City. He had lost my mother to pancreatic cancer over a decade earlier, but he had sustained an active social and intellectual life. He had three daughters who lived close by with their families. He had eight grandchildren who adored him. Every year or so, he would travel to Europe and stay in his favorite little hotels in Paris, London, and Berlin with various side trips to scout out some new destination. He passionately loved Henry James and Anthony Trollope. He was a scholar of Thomas Jefferson. He had been turned down for an interview with the CIA because, after graduating from college in 1949—and on the GI bill—he had once given a dollar to the Communist Party, something his mother-in-law held against him until the day she died. He mixed an exceptionally strong martini. His health was robust, except for mild type 2 diabetes, which he developed in his seventies and controlled through his diet.

In the late summer of 2006, he suddenly developed double vision. On the advice of his eye doctor, Dad went to see Dr. H, the chair of the Ophthalmology Department at a major teaching hospital in the city. Although Dad's diabetes was discussed in the preliminary consultation, Dr. H zeroed in on the possibility of a very rare, but potentially devastating disorder: temporal arteritis, an inflammation of an artery that runs along the temple. Temporal arteritis, if left untreated, can lead to stroke or blindness. A biopsy—the only way to confirm the diagnosis—was scheduled for early the following week. To prevent inflammation, Dad was to begin taking 100 mg of prednisone daily, a routinely prescribed corticosteroid, although, as we learned only later, in an unusually high dose.

While filling the prescription, the head pharmacist at the hospital came out to express his concern that the dose was so high. He asked Dad to please check with Dr. H before starting the medication. My father did not want to "question" the chairman of a department and did not act on the pharmacist's advice. Too many patients are reticent about questioning doctors, especially the more credentialed they are. But as we were soon to find out, a lapse in clear, simple communication between doctor and patient can lead to devastating consequences.

Dad started the medication that day. He and my sister Martha, who accompanied him when he saw Dr. H, had never discussed anything during the exam about the medication dosage or possible side effects. Dad just took the medicine—unaware that at a very high dosage he put himself at greater risk for its most severe side effects, including mania, psychosis, and heart failure. Additionally, he was never informed that corticosteroids cause immediate and sometimes severe elevation of blood sugar levels in people with diabetes. Typically, if a diabetic is prescribed steroid therapy there is a plan in place to monitor blood sugar levels daily because of this potentially deadly side effect. We did not know any of this then; we didn't ask and we weren't told. Dad was just another typically passive patient in the "don't ask, don't tell" routine taking place every day in rushed doctor/patient consultations across this country. Patients don't ask basic questions about prescriptions and side effects—assuming, I guess, that they will be told if there are any. But in not asking, patients avoid taking responsibility for their own health—a magic pill will cure everything, even if you don't really know why you are taking it. Does anyone ever actually read the drug inserts that accompany prescriptions? No, because they seem to be written in ancient Greek and they're generally printed in tiny type. Nor do most people want to trouble the harried pharmacist for basic information about the drugs they are about to ingest. And doctors, for their part, fail to communicate—in terms a layperson can understand—why you need a medication, what it does, and precisely how to take it.

My family did not know that medication errors are responsible for 28 percent of all hospital admissions, according to a *New York Times* article. If listed as such, it would be the fifth leading cause of death in the United States. Americans are taking more and more medication without adequately understanding why. In fact, 66 percent of all adults in the United States use prescription drugs; one-third take five or more medications every day. My family's passivity and ignorance about prescription medication played a role in making Dad literally crazy almost overnight.

The biopsy showed no blockage, but vaguely written post-op instructions to "continue all pre-op medications" led Dad to believe he was to continue the steroids, since that was the only medication he was taking before surgery. With outpatient surgery, it can be especially disorienting for the patient to be woken up from anesthesia, handed post-op instructions while barely conscious, and hustled out of the recovery room door still groggy and groaning with pain. Dad had not discussed post-op care with his doctor before surgery—another serious lapse in essential doctor/patient communication. He stumbled home from surgery and continued to take the steroids.

When I am telling a doctor this story, it is at this juncture that he or she will invariably ask, "And how soon was it before your dad went crazy?" Not long. Before the double vision had even cropped up, Dad had been planning a trip to his house in Virginia, just to check on a few things. After the biopsy, with his double vision still unresolved, my sisters and I figured the trip was definitely off. But Dad was insistent on driving down to Virginia—two days after his surgery. His plans had also expanded slightly from meeting with a new handyman and gardener to planning a gigantic eighty-second birthday party for himself to be held in Virginia. My sisters and I were horrified, first and foremost, at the thought of an ailing eighty-one-year-old with double vision behind the wheel of a moving car. Also, the party idea seemed a little weird, since we all live in New York City. After much negotiation, we got him to agree to call his eye doctor and get an okay to make the four-hundred-mile trip—certain that would be the end of any road trips for the foreseeable future. Incredibly, Dr. H simply suggested that Dad drive with one eye closed to counter the double vision—for four hundred miles! Dad triumphantly and maniacally started planning his four-hundred-mile one-eyed journey. The next day, I stopped by his apartment in a last-ditch effort to talk him out of going. I found him frantically rearranging thirty grocery bags filled with Spam, Mallomars, and toilet paper. When I asked what was going on, he replied, "Isn't it obvious these items are essential to my survival?" Where he really needed my help was to figure out a way to fit a gigantic dresser from his bedroom into the front seat of his car—a task akin to stuffing an NBA basketball player into a baby seat on the back of a bike. He simply did not have time to explain why he needed that dresser in Virginia.

Suddenly, he burst into tears as he clutched my hands and told me he was overwhelmed by so many important world-saving ideas and the lack of time to implement them all, let alone the time to simply tell them all to somebody, anybody. I snuck into the hallway to phone my sisters to sound the alarm that Dad had gone suddenly and completely crazy. I didn't know how or why it had happened, but there was a lunatic in his living room and it wasn't our father.

None of us could fathom what was going on. We never

thought about the steroid medication—although at this point Dad was carrying it around in a baggie like a junkie. I had taken prednisone a few times in the past for sun poisoning. It always got rid of the rash and, at the time, I didn't seem crazier than usual. Of course, I had taken just a fraction of what Dad was ingesting on a daily basis.

My sisters and I held on to the magical thinking that a good night's sleep would make everything go back to normal. The three of us formulated a plan: my sister Martha and I would go to Dad's apartment the next morning before he was to leave to tag-team him so that he would postpone his trip either from exhaustion or exasperation. Martha, always his favorite, could be the reasonable, lawyerly negotiator—the understanding good cop. I would be the complete skeptic—the bad cop in the corner repeating, "This is nuts," over and over again.

Wouldn't you know it, when we got to Dad's building at seven o'clock in the morning, he had already finished loading his '76 Caprice with the help of his politely incredulous doorman—as if he had anticipated our carefully planned showdown. The bags of Spam were piled from floor to ceiling in the backseat, blocking his rearview mirror. The trunk was filled with as many of his books as he could fit, as well as a tuxedo he had not worn in twenty-five years and his patent-leather dress shoes—perhaps in anticipation of that birthday party. He had the dresser out on the sidewalk, but after a few futile attempts, even he had to grudgingly admit that there was no way it could possibly fit in the front seat. Instead, he decided to load the seat with a few shopping bags of random but quite necessary things like old lamps, shoe polish, and various silver serving pieces.

Behind Dad's back, I was waving my arms at Martha and silently shrieking, "Dad has gone nuts!" and "Call 911!" Martha tried the calm approach at dissuasion while furtively hissing at me that we did not have a legal leg to stand on to prevent Dad from getting behind the wheel, now that he had a doctor's clearance. He brushed aside her entreaties with the parting words that he needed to get going because he was going to throw himself the biggest birthday party southwest Virginia had ever seen. The elderly guy driving away with one eye closed and a car filled with Spam had somehow managed to steal the body and soul of the erudite, gentlemanly, slightly fantasy-prone father we knew.

Within hours, he was lost on the highways heading south, even though he had made that trip hundreds of times. Two days later, we finally caught up with him after he called us from a motel in Virginia. The next morning, back in New York, Dad was in the emergency room of Dr. H's hospital, suffering from full-blown steroid-induced psychosis. Dad, quite simply, had gone completely crazy from a routinely prescribed medication. A cascading series of breakdowns in basic doctor/patient communication had led to a medical catastrophe.

Until that moment in the emergency room, Dad had never spent a night in a hospital—except during World War II. In addition to suffering from steroid-induced psychosis, his blood sugar had shot up to diabetic coma–inducing levels. The emergency room doctors surmised that it had actually been a slowly rising blood sugar level over the past several months that caused his double vision—a common symptom when diabetes gets out of control. The steroids basically acted like a nuclear bomb on his endocrine system as well as his psyche. He had never needed to take the steroids; his blood sugar levels should have been checked early on to see if there was a systemic reason for his double vision. In addition, he should never have continued taking them after surgery, but his post-op instructions were unclear.

For the next month, Dad was a patient at one of the top hospitals in the country. He not only had Medicare but also supplemental AARP insurance. My two sisters and I and our families all lived close by. As a family, we thought we had the resources—financial, educational, and professional—to safely guide Dad through his hospital stay.

We were wrong.

Patients who enter a hospital today have no idea what they will confront until already trapped in the trenches: the frantic pace, the fragmented care by a rotating cast of doctors and stressed-out nurses, an endless series of treatments and medications without adequate explanation or oversight, and simply not enough face time with their health-care team, upon whom they are so dependent. Being sick in the hospital is a strange, frightening, and lonely experience made even more overwhelming by the absence of simple compassion—the human connection even in a sea of busy people. Hospital staff can all seem too busy to help you.

During this first hospitalization—for it was to become the first of many—seven different doctors as well as numerous nameless residents and interns treated Dad. Each physician focused solely on his particular specialty—Dad's diabetes, his heart, his mind, and so on. Tracking the medications, tests, and treatments that each doctor prescribed for specific problems was confounding. Trying to glean a morsel of information from any of the doctors on their different rounds was next to impossible. The doctors seemed to have an unerring sense of knowing exactly when to drop in on Dad: just as the sleeping pill was taking effect or when one of us had run out for a much-needed coffee break. There was an enormous information vacuum—so many doctors but so little time to connect and communicate. The most immediate medical issue for Dad was to get his blood sugar under control. He was put on insulin injections for the first time and a highly restricted salt- and sugar-free diet. For our family, however, the most frightening issue was not his biological disorder—but whether our dad would ever return to the person we knew.

Small mistakes in the most routine aspects of his care began to multiply on a daily basis. At least once a day, Dad was given the wrong food—orange juice, pancakes, and maple syrup for breakfast, for instance, even though his endocrinologist stressed how important it was to be vigilant in monitoring Dad's dietary restrictions, particularly his sugar intake. It slowly dawned on us that one of us had to be there at all mealtimes to check his tray. Fortunately, Dad in his mania thought the dietetic hospital food could give his favorite restaurants competition for their Zagat's stars. Sugar-free gelatin that tasted "so wonderful" was one of the few fringe benefits of his psychosis.

Dad was on a daily regimen of many pills, as well as insulin injections. He would get six to eight pills in a little paper cup several times a day. Initially, our family had only the vaguest understanding of what he was taking, why he was taking it, and who prescribed it. We trusted the system. It was only after we began to notice pills on the floor or in his bed that we realized no one was monitoring his medications. Dad had so many small pills to take, but his hands were large and his fingers stiff. It was just too easy for Dad to drop a pill as he tried to steer it to his mouth and too easy for the staff to simply not notice. How was it affecting his recovery if a scheduled antipsychotic medication or heart medicine wound up under his bed or in his covers and no one knew?

CEOs of hospitals don't seem to understand that it is the relentless absence of even the smallest sympathetic gesture, coupled with the accumulation of oversights, that ultimately drives patients and families crazy. Dad would go for an MRI and then be left to wait for hours, in a wheelchair in a busy hallway with other barely clothed patients, for someone—anyone—to return him to his room. It was only after Dad got fed up with the humiliating wait and started to wheel himself furiously toward the elevators—with loud running commentary—that a nurse came racing from somewhere and summoned an aide to take him back to his room. Every day you felt just a little bit more demoralized and dehumanized.

To the hospital staff, Dad was just another patient. To us, his family, who knew him as he had been before, he was, indeed, sometimes an annoying, crazy old man. We never forgot that he wound up in the hospital because of a medication error, but the daily grind of hospital life didn't make it easy for those of us who knew and loved him as he was before this catastrophe. Little by little we realized, as a family, that we had a responsibility to resist the cloak of anonymity. We also realized that we were left on our own to piece together our individual observations and whatever bits of information we managed to glean from various doctors or nurses. There did not seem to be one clear, concise, overall hospital plan for care. Daily, Dad swung very high and very low. He wrestled with horrific flashbacks from his World War II service in the Pacific—a time he had never discussed with anyone. These memories seemed to crop up mostly at night. In the mornings, he often obsessed about painful childhood memories growing up during the Depression. By late morning, he would flip into a giddy mania where he would busily plan a cocktail party in his room so his friends could admire his seventeenth-floor view of the East River!

The longer a loved one is in the hospital, the greater the likelihood that a straw will break the camel's back and turn a semi-meek family member into a radicalized patient advocate. For me, it was the Saturday afternoon I arrived at the hospital to discover that Dad had been missing for several hours—and no one on the hospital staff even knew it.

It was the only day all of us had taken the morning to catch up with our own family affairs. I couldn't get to the hospital until 2 p.m. Dad was not in his room, but I noticed an untouched lunch tray. Since by that point I had been tracking his meal schedule, I knew his lunch had been delivered around 11:30 a.m. An untouched lunch tray meant that he had not eaten in at least two and a half hours. It also might mean he had not been given his premeal insulin shot—a terrifying situation, given his diabetes. No one on the staff had noticed that he was gone, even though his room was directly across from the nurses' station.

After I searched the hospital with security guards, my sister Mary-Paula tried calling Dad's apartment. No one thought he could possibly be there—he had no money for one thing—and it was so far away. But he answered his phone. It was the weekend, when a hospital can seem like a ghost town with a skeleton staff. He had given the guards in the empty lobby a friendly wave goodbye, his hospital bracelet dangling from his wrist. He wore a crazy combination of his own clothes and a hospital gown. He took a taxi to his apartment and borrowed cab fare from his doorman, since he didn't have his wallet. The doorman noted the time—11 a.m.—because Dad was weaving through the lobby as if he were drunk. (Diabetics can become disoriented and unsteady if they are getting into trouble with their blood sugar levels.)

We realized that by the time we finally found Dad, he had been gone from the hospital for over six hours. He had missed two rounds of insulin, all his other medications, and one meal. When Mary-Paula spoke to him, though, he cheerfully said he had spent a wonderful afternoon in his bedroom catching butterflies with a giant net. He had found a can of baked beans to eat in an otherwise empty kitchen.

Two days after Dad's great escape, the hospital came to us and said that since his blood sugar levels were suddenly under control, Medicare would no longer pay for him to remain in a regular hospital room as he was "medically stable." The steroid-induced psychosis was another matter. We had two options: we could take him home and hire around-the-clock untrained health aides to care for him at $4,500 a week (not covered by Medicare), or we could commit him to the hospital's psych ward.

(Note to families: check with your insurance company directly to see what your coverage is. Also, every hospital has a mechanism that allows a patient to appeal a discharge he or she feels is too early. We didn't know any of this.) We thought he needed rest and quiet—and some measure of control. He was still trying to unionize the hospital orderlies, dressing down the arrogant young residents, and working on a plan to remodel all the hospital bathrooms. We had never seen a psych ward before. I envisioned long, erudite conversations with a psychiatrist interspersed with quiet hours in a book-filled library. Dad carefully read his voluntary commitment form and went over the finer legal points with a hospital representative. When he was first wheeled into his Spartan new room—a single bed, a desk, a chair, and an overhead light—he said, "I always wanted to have a quiet room like this." It was only as we were leaving him that we really noticed the unnatural quiet, the heightened sense of loneliness, and the silent, expressionless, medicated patients sitting alone in their rooms.

An extremely young resident and a nurse conducted his intake. We discussed Dad's very restricted diet—especially no orange juice, as it would send his blood sugar soaring. We reminded them that he had always led an independent life and was an early-to-bed, early-to-rise kind of guy. They assured us that they accommodated patients' temperaments and habits. We also discussed Dad's World War II memories, which were causing him such suffering. As if on cue, he launched into a horrific tale of being on Guam and suffering a migraine as his Marine platoon was inching on their bellies to higher ground. Dad had been all of nineteen at the time. At nightfall, he and his buddy dug a small hollow. They could hear snipers all around them. Dad, because of a terrible migraine, was throwing up all night into his helmet, terrified that his being sick would get his buddy killed. It was obvious how much Dad was suffering—suffering from the steroids still in his system, suffering from long-suppressed memories, suffering because he was a human being who was ill. The young resident listened to him with a stony blank face.

The next day, my sister Mary-Paula and I went to visit Dad during the highly restricted visiting hours. Dad was not in his room. When we asked for him at the nurses' station, everyone got that deer-in-the-headlights look. The stony-faced young resident appeared and ushered us into a little side office. She began by saying there had been an "incident" with Dad, but he was resting now—in lockdown, shackled to a metal gurney, shot full of enough antipsychotic medication to subdue a horse.

Apparently, Dad had been "difficult" in the early morning. He had gotten up at 5 a.m. to shower and get dressed. The nurses ordered him back to bed, although we had told them he had been getting up at 5 a.m. for the past forty years. I am sure Dad was looking forward to a nice cup of coffee and the *New York Times*—not a SWAT team.

He got back into his hospital gown but decided the psych ward was for the birds. He wrote out a legal notice that he wanted to be released. Since he had voluntarily committed himself, he thought that was all he needed to do and was free to go. He packed his little rollaway suitcase and got dressed. He dropped off his legal request for release at the nurses' station—just as late-morning snacks of orange juice and muffins were being handed out to all the patients, including Dad. Thirty minutes later, he put on his hat and blazer and prepared to leave, no doubt with elevated blood sugar levels. Alarms went off and four guards were called.

When Dad saw the guards, he reminded them that he was a U.S. Marine and they would never take him alive. They wrestled my eighty-one-year-old dad to the floor, stripped him in front of the other patients, and took him to the "quiet room." I think there were a total of fourteen patients in the psychiatric wing when Dad was there, but no one seemed to think it was important to call the family—especially the stony-faced young resident.

After that traumatic event, our family focused on getting him out of the psych ward as soon as we could care for him safely at home. But once again we were unable to make a plan with any help from the hospital staff. And, again, on several occasions we found his antipsychotic medications on the floor. The hospital finally assigned an aide to help him take his medications, since, with such restricted visiting hours, we could not be there each time he was due to take his medicine. Yet in all this time we never met with a case manager or social worker to help organize his care. I am an inveterate list maker. The value of checklists was made apparent to me in my professional life as a producer, director, and head of music-video production for two major music labels. My checklists were essential for organizing the many details of multiple music-video productions—usually with overlapping production schedules. On any given film shoot, there are hundreds of things that need to be coordinated and thus hundreds of things that can go wrong. Each film project is unique—different musical artists, directors, crews, budgets, locations, technical requirements, and creative goals—yet each production requires the coordination of many people from multiple departments with a variety of technical and creative skills (camera, set design, lighting, grip, wardrobe, etc.) working together within a very limited amount of time to create something that you hope has that little bit of film magic.

Necessity is the mother of invention—or adaptation at the very least. In the hospital, I often felt as if I were on some crazy film set. Consider the sheer number of people involved in typical patient care—from the orderly to the superspecialist; the constant flood of incoming information; our reliance on technology and, with it, complicated equipment and machinery; the constant time pressure to get things done now; and the intense mix of personalities and emotions. Yes, I thought, as I stood in the hospital hallway one day, I could see how I could put my producer skills—and especially my checklists—to work to help us manage Dad's hospital stay. I began to adapt my film production checklists to the demands of "hospital production" for Dad—to organize this complex situation into manageable details to ensure things got done and, in doing so, protect him first as a person and then as a patient.

All patients need to organize for themselves the overwhelming amount of information, treatments, and personnel that they will encounter during a hospital stay. Every patient's situation is different and all hospitals are different, but the fundamental care protocols, from your perspective as a patient, remain the same—getting information so you can understand and agree to your treatment, monitoring your care, collaborating with your doctors and nurses, making yourself as comfortable and safe as possible, and making sure you are being heard—in short, becoming an active partner with your health-care team.

My family needed a user-friendly system, in one easy-to-reference book, to organize Dad's daily care immediately. We needed a family hospital production guide similar to my film production notebook. Without such a book, we found ourselves always scrambling to piece together various scribbled notes and bits of information, which was proving to be a woefully inadequate approach to managing his care.

In my preliminary research for this book, I happened upon an article in the *New Yorker* by Atul Gawande, the surgeon and writer, about the work of Dr. Peter Pronovost, from Johns Hopkins Medical Center, who developed a checklist program for health-care workers to use in intensive care units to lower infection rates. Dr. Pronovost instituted a simple five-step checklist to reduce the possibility of hospital-acquired infections when inserting a central venous catheter—a common necessity in the

ICU. The first step on the checklist calls for health-care workers to wash their hands with soap. This seems shockingly obvious to the layperson, but after spending so much time in different hospitals, I know firsthand how often the basics—handwashing, correct dosage of medications, meal delivery to the right patient, removing an IV or catheter as soon as possible under sterile conditions—slip through the cracks in the overall hospital chaos.

The hospitals that implemented Dr. Pronovost's simple five-step checklist reduced their catheter infection rate to zero! The documented success of Dr. Pronovost's simple checklist encouraged me that checklists could be helpful for patients and their family and friends. Checklists provide a simple framework to start to make sense of the enormous amount of information a patient receives. Checklists help you translate medical jargon into plain language—understandable, human-size units of information—so you can be more proactive during a hospital stay.

As a producer, my production team always reviewed our "idiot" checklist the night before every shoot. Did we have what we need? Did we overlook anything? Did we pick up the film or give the crew the right call times to be on set? We also checked to make sure we had what we needed to get that complex technical shot. I didn't have to know how to make the car crash happen—but I had to make sure we had the best stunt crew, the best technical plan and equipment, and the appropriate safety measures in place. Most important, I needed to make sure everyone was on the same page. A small mistake can be corrected; a cascade of small errors leads to big problems. I knew my production checklists could be adapted to help families organize a loved one's care—their hospital production—and help prevent the feeling of constantly careening around one hairpin turn after another—without the benefit of a stunt driver's expertise.

Too often, life involves planned and unplanned trips to the

hospital. Illness and injury are a part of every human experience. Over the past decade, I have used and adapted my checklists to advocate for many patients during their hospital stays. I have learned, through a lot of hard-earned experience, to be a better, more organized advocate by using simple checklists to keep track of complex hospital care. I now know that once patients enter a hospital for treatment of any kind, what they need most of all is information—what is happening to them and why. As for my Dad—whose story began my long journey into patient advocacy—he was deemed "cured" and discharged by the hospital. But he was never fully himself again, never "whole." My sisters and I became his daily caregivers for the last decade of his life. He finally found some peace, and a belonging, when I transferred all of his health care to the VA near his apartment. The other vets gave him back his dignity by saluting him every time he walked into the hospital wearing his WWII Marine cap. By the end of his life, what mattered most to him was being able to read the *New York Times* from cover to cover, enjoy a bowl of vanilla ice cream, and drink his treasured gin martini. When he could no longer enjoy those, he just turned his face toward the morning sun streaming through the window and died peacefully in the hospice unit at the VA hospital. This time, at his final leave taking from a hospital, a young soldier stood at attention as they wheeled his body down the hall and then began to play taps.

The ten simple checklists in this book can help you handle the realities of present-day hospital patient care in this country. Hopefully, these checklists will be a daily reminder to patients and families that each of us must play a big role in ensuring two crucial aspects of quality patient care: guarding against simple human error that can derail the best care and promoting simple human kindness to ensure that patients are not only "cured" but also "healed" in the wholeness of their being.

If the simple phrase "person first, patient second" becomes

your mantra during a hospital stay, it will remind you to protect, support, and value your whole being and not succumb to the hospital's tendency to reduce you to an organ, a diagnosis, a surgical procedure . . . in other words, just another anonymous patient.

Introduction

More than 36 million Americans are admitted to the hospital each year. If you are reading this book, you or someone you love is probably one of these patients. All patients need help in understanding what is happening to them during a complicated, often dangerous, and always lonely journey through our modern American hospital system.

I address *you* in this introduction and throughout the book, but it is always the collective *you* of patient, family, and friends who must come together to weather any individual's health crisis. Many of the suggestions in this book go beyond the capacity or capability of sick patients who may not be conscious of what is going on around them much of the time. Some patients have limited tolerance for how much medical information they can and want to process and would prefer to leave partnering with their care team to their family. Some are children or a frail parent who are entirely dependent on you to safely navigate them through a hospital stay. This book provides guidance to help you—the collective *you*—family who are friends or friends who are family to harness your resources, individually and as a group or team, to obtain the safest possible care.

First, remember that friends and family possess critical knowledge of the patient as a human being with a history—a life not defined by illness or injury. The person comes first, the patient second. Consequently, a family's observations about a loved one make a tremendous, though often overlooked, contribution to planning and assessing treatment. You are the ones who know what is normal—the baseline—for the patient in their daily life. The individual's story is as important as scientific data in judging if treatment is actually working. Every individual is unique and responds uniquely, no matter how standardized the treatment. Family can provide an invaluable and coequal perspective along with the hospital team in gauging the effectiveness of treatment. Combining your understanding of the patient as a whole person with a daily checklist to monitor the medical details of treatment can make you a powerful advocate for your loved one.

All patients and their family need a basic road map to navigate the confusing and intimidating terrain of any hospital. Too often, patients and their family, with so much at stake, can feel as if they are careening down an endless road, punctuated by too many high-tech procedures and treatments, too many medications, too much incomplete information absent the fundamental way-finding tool: clear and meaningful communication with their health-care team.

This book provides a series of simple checklists to help you, the person, now a patient, bridge the gap between your expectations for and the reality of getting safe, attentive, and compassionate care during a hospital stay. These checklists have distilled the best evidence based resources and research into a user-friendly, easy-to-organize system to help you better manage, monitor, and participate in your hospital care.

These ten simple checklists are devised to help you accomplish two key goals. The first is to get the information you need to make informed choices about your care. The checklists help you collect, organize, and get a better handle on both the big picture and the critical routine daily details involved in your care. The second is to provide a constant reminder of the primacy of the "person." You. What are your wishes, choices, and hopes for treatment? Medical care is an intricate, highly technical dance, but you are the essential partner with your doctor. Information sharing is vital to safe, optimal care.

The first thing you must understand is that you do not need to know how to perform your own surgery, insert an IV, take an x-ray, read a CT scan, draw blood, or perform any other medical procedure in order to better protect your safety and enhance your care. However you do need to:

1. Understand *why* every single action is being done to your body, you, in the hospital.
2. Agree that every action is *necessary* and *appropriate* treatment for you.
3. Be sure that every single detail of treatment—no matter how routine—is being done under *sanitary* conditions, using best practices, and is meant for *you*.

When you are well, it is all too easy to be lulled into complacency and passivity by the magical thinking that a hospital is the institutional version of your mother nursing you back to health: comfort and compassion in perfect harmony with medical art and scientific technology; the reassuring hand on the forehead coupled with an MRI; an unhurried and caring bedside manner complementing brilliant diagnostic and surgical skill. A patient hopes for state-of-the-art yet humane and attentive treatment—the miraculous dovetailing with the mundane.

The reality of hospital care is altogether different.

Consider these statistics:

- A hospital patient, on average, is subject to one medication error per day.
- Every six minutes a patient dies in an American hospital from a hospital-acquired infection, an infection acquired after admission and that is usually the result of poor hand hygiene.
- Sixty-five percent of identified adverse patient events—that is, an unintended medical event that causes serious harm to or death of a patient—were found to have communication failures as the underlying root cause.

There are fifty million surgical procedures performed every year in the United States. There are thousands of different medications and treatments to consider for a multitude of possible diagnoses. Doctors and nurses are responsible for increasingly complex care of growing numbers of patients, each confronting a health crisis—a life crisis. These frontline health-care professionals always want to deliver the best possible care, but their ability to do so both depends on and is hampered by a vast, invisible hospital infrastructure of hundreds of separate departments—labs, pharmacies, medical records, and so on. Under the best of circumstances, mistakes in medical care can be made because doctors and nurses (or the lab technician, radiologist, or pharmacist you never see) are fallible; they are human. Given the frantic pace and fragmented care in today's technology-driven hospitals, mistakes in communication and lack of careful attention to detail are not just likely, they are inevitable, and the consequence all too often is patient harm.

This book's ten commonsense checklists encourage you to ask questions about all aspects of your hospital care. By familiarizing yourself with your medical situation, you will be a better watchdog and advocate for yourself. Every patient needs to think about these essential questions:

- What is going in and out of my body today? And why?
- What is the reason each of my medications has been prescribed and by whom? Is it the right dose, the right schedule, the right patient—me?
- How does the surgical site feel and look?
- Are my IVs and other invasive devices, such as catheters, drains, or breathing tubes, monitored frequently to make sure everything is working okay and there are no infections? When can they be removed?—ask that question every day.
- Why has my treatment plan changed? Who ordered the change? Did I agree to the change after it was discussed with me?
- Do all my health-care providers wash their hands before they touch me, change an IV, hand me medication, deliver my food, or do anything else that involves direct contact?
- Do I know the names of everyone on my care team?
- Who is in charge of my overall care—a hospitalist and not my surgeon or specialist?
- When is the handoff (shift change) for all the members of my hospital team? How do they accurately relate all information about my current status and care plan to the new staff coming on?
- Are the daily goals of care my goals?

Like it or not, *you* are the one constant in your hospital stay, confined to your bed as doctors and nurses examine you, dispense medications, check monitors, take your vitals, and perform any number of other tasks. Only by being engaged and alert can you (the collective *you*) get safer, better care by short-circuiting the main causes of preventable medical error:

- When communication breaks down between patient and doctor, between family and doctors, between doctors and nurses, and between doctors themselves.
- When safe, sanitary practices fall by the wayside.
- When mistakes happen because of human error with the details of care—a medication oversight, a wrong code entered in the computer while adding chart notes, a failure to pass along key information at shift changes.

Hospital staff rarely have the time to be concerned with comfort issues that are essential to true healing and full recovery. Friends and family must take the lead in providing comfort and compassion—as integral to healing the human being as medical treatment is to curing the ailment. The checklists provide suggestions for family and friends to improve a patient's quality of life at this most crucial time by giving equal weight to the importance of high touch and not just high-tech care.

The single greatest threat to a patient's safety in hospitals is simple human error: communication breakdowns stemming from overly fragmented care by overworked doctors and nurses, lapses in the most basic sanitary practices, and mistakes in routine care because of the frantic hospital pace.

The single greatest threat to a patient's sanity in the hospital is the dehumanizing and demoralizing atmosphere that pervades our modern medical institutions. At your sickest and most vulnerable, you may feel profoundly alone because of the absence of essential human connection amid the flurry of tests and treatments and an array of largely anonymous hospital staff.

The checklists in this book can help make your journey from person to patient and back again safer and saner by helping you to better advocate for yourself as a person first and a patient second.

How to Use the Checklists

Good checklists . . . are efficient, to the point, and easy to use in the most difficult situations. They do not try to spell out everything. Instead, they provide reminders of only the most critical and important steps. They are, above all, practical.

—Atul Gawande, *The Checklist Manifesto*

Each checklist partners with the others, loops back and revisits important information, offers continual reminders to track details, prompts you to ask questions and trust your intuition because your voice matters in a hospital room.

The Patient's Checklist is:
- A user-friendly and efficient step-by-step action plan to help you and your family organize complicated medical information.
- A series of prompts to remind you to be vigilant about monitoring and managing the critical details of day-to-day

7

patient care in a busy hospital setting so you don't have to rely on your memory alone.

- A way to promote collaboration and communication between you, your family, your doctors, and your nurses about your goals of care that are key to promoting patient safety and achieving better outcomes.
- An up-to-the-minute daily record of your hospital stay. You create your own patient medical and information flowchart—a layperson's version of the one used by your nurses and doctors.
- An invaluable reminder to protect the needs, wishes, choices, and hopes of the person who has the most at stake in a health crisis—the patient.

Checklist Summaries

Checklist 1: Before You Go

The foundation. This first list prepares you for the journey and shows you how to be a more informed, prepared, and proactive patient. You'll ask questions, you'll gather your team to help you share the burden of your care, you'll supply guidance to your loved ones. This list outlines the first steps in active partnering with your clinical team—they work as a team, so can you and your family.

Checklist 2: What to Bring

The practical and the personal. This list underscores things to bring to help you hold on to your humanity, sanity, and safety in the impersonal and chaotic world of a hospital.

Checklist 3: During Your Stay

The big picture. This list shares practical suggestions for ways to increase your comfort during your hospital stay and partner effectively with everyone on your care team to get better, safer care.

Checklist 4: Master Medication List

The overview. This list offers an easy-to-understand, comprehensive guide to your prescribed medications during your entire hospital stay. By filling in this easy-to-use chart you will familiarize yourself with what your meds actually look like, why you are taking them, and the overall schedule for taking them.

Checklist 5: Daily Medication Log

The details. A daily log to make sure that every time medication is given to you it is the right drug, the right dose, the right schedule, the right method (that is, by mouth, by injection, etc.)—and that it is meant for you!

Checklist 6: Daily Journal

The progress report. This lists provides a journal, with a daily checklist, to help you chronicle everything that happens to you while you're in the hospital.

Checklist 7: Discharge Plan

The transition. Leaving the hospital for home or rehab is a time of relief but also a time that requires great care. Here you'll find tips to help plan for your discharge from the moment you enter the hospital, with a focus on education, getting needs met, referrals, and therapeutic and social services beyond the hospital so you can recover safely and avoid readmission.

Checklist 8: Insurance

Suggestions to help organize what will become the huge challenge of navigating our insurance system.

Checklist 9: Doctor Contacts

Provides a contact list to organize everyone on your hospital care team as well as discharge referrals and vendors.

Checklist 10: Family & Friends Contacts

Consolidates all the contact information for the important people in your life who are helping you navigate this hospital stay.

Before You Go

"It is important that we all be active decision makers in medical treatment, because medical decisions will have a powerful influence on our bodies and on our lives. That is why medical decisions are fundamentally personal decisions: different people place different values on longevity, functioning, risk, and appearance."

—George J. Annas, *The Rights of Patients*

Family members of hospitalized patients play a vital role in detecting signs of deterioration in patient health status, which helps prevent further clinical deterioration. They are often more familiar with the patient's behavior and health history and better in detecting slight changes in a patient's health status.

JBI Database of Systematic Reviews and Implementation Reports 12, no. 9 (2014): 58–68

Between 210,000–440,000 patients each year who go to the hospital for care suffer some type of preventable harm that contributes to their death.

Journal of Patient Safety 9, no. 3 (2013): 122–128C

Practical Steps to Prepare for a Hospital Stay

☐ 1. Ask yourself this central question: *Who will be my support system while I am in the hospital?*

- Having involved family and friends at your bedside is the single most important way to ensure better, safer care within the busy, complicated world of any hospital.
- A support system can monitor your routine daily care.
- Involved family and friends can keep lines of communication open with your hospital care team.
- A support system offers you comfort in the cold and sterile environment of the hospital.
- Because they know you in your everyday life, your family and friends can provide much needed information to your doctors and nurses about your normal baseline—what is the "normal" you against which any recovery needs to be assessed.
- Your family and friends are your best advocates.

☐ 2. Think back on any previous experiences with hospitalizations—either your own or those of a parent, sibling, other family member, friend, work colleague, and so on—what were the lessons learned?

- What went wrong and what went right?
- These takeaways can help you clarify your own concerns, fears, hopes, and preferences for treatment based on your current medical situation and form the basis for discussion with your family about your personal *goals of care*.
- "Goals of care" is a term your medical team may use a lot. To your medical team, the goals of care are oriented toward the body and improving function by correcting

or removing impairment. To you, the patient, your goals of care are about what's most important to you, your values, your wishes. How you personally see the risks and benefits of any medical decision should be the defining factor in choosing a pathway.

- The more your family understands what you would want or do not want with your personal goals of care, the more informed they will be and the better able they will be to advocate for you and engage effectively as partners with your hospital care team.

3. **Choose a medical decision maker and sign a health-care proxy form now.**

- Every person should designate a health-care proxy—also known, in plain language, as a medical or health-care decision maker—preferably when you are well! It is not necessary to wait to until you are actually a patient to complete this important health document. Accidents and illness are an unpredictable fact of life.

- If you don't formally designate a health-care proxy, often those closest to you and who know you best will not be allowed to help make critical medical decisions for you.

- Your proxy can be anyone you trust—your spouse, partner, friend, adult child, or sibling, for instance—and with whom you have discussed your preferences for your medical treatment in the event you are unable to make those decisions for yourself.

- You are not signing away your rights! The role of the health-care proxy is only in effect if and when you are so sick that you cannot speak for yourself.

- Health-care proxies are legally empowered to play an active role in your care decisions and can make sure hospitals and doctors follow your wishes.

- Your proxy has a legal right to access your medical record to help make decisions for you.
- Every state has its own official form, which is easy to download and fill out. See the Resources section at the end of this book.
- Keep a hard copy for yourself and give copies to your health-care proxy and your primary care doctor, if you have one.
- Take a photo or scan the completed document to store on your phone too.
- Share your health-care proxy choice now with other family members and friends to prevent any confusion later on. Give them copies if you want to.
- Make sure the hospital knows who your medical decision maker is and adds your completed health-care proxy form to your hospital chart.
- If you have not filled out a health-care proxy form before admission—especially if it is an unanticipated visit to the ER—all hospitals have this important document available for patients and will help you to complete it.

4. **Create a living will, which is a different but complementary advance directive to your health-care proxy.**
- There is a difference between having a health-care proxy and having a living will.
- Your health-care proxy is the person you have chosen to make medical decisions for you when you are unable to do so. A living will is the opportunity for you to describe what kinds of life-sustaining medical interventions—things like a ventilator (breathing machine), artificial nutrition (feeding tube), resuscitation (CPR and other interventions)—you want and

for how long if you become terminally ill and/or permanently incapacitated. A living will also specifies when or if you would want palliative care, also known as comfort care.

- These two documents complement each other and are like having insurance for your home—you hope you won't need them but having them offers precious guidance *from you* to your family, your appointed health-care proxy, and your medical team about what really matters to you.
- A living will is not a legal document like a health-care proxy, but it is a written record that spells out to your family and your health-care team which medical treatments you do or do not want.
- An alternative to a written living will is to record a video on your phone explaining what you do and do not want in the event that you cannot speak for yourself. If you do this, share it with your family members.
- The important point is that a living will gives you the opportunity to make known to your family, your best advocates, what matters most to you.
- See Resources for websites that provide in-depth information on various advance directive forms and conversation starter kits that can be very helpful.

☐ 5. Pick a family spokesperson.

- It is extremely helpful for a patient and family to choose one family spokesperson if many are involved in your care. Doctors and nurses simply do not have the time to field multiple phone calls from different family members.
- Your family spokesperson is the communication bridge between the hospital team and the family. This

person should be a good listener as they will be the point person for medical updates from your doctors and nurses. Your spokesperson also needs to be good at listening to and communicating the questions and concerns that other family members may have.

- Your spokesperson can be your medical decision maker but doesn't have to be. For instance, perhaps your spouse or partner is your medical decision maker, but an adult child or a sibling may be the right choice as the family spokesperson.

- As with COVID-19, in the future all hospitals may contend with periodic isolation policies or other situations in which visitors are severely restricted. You and your family need a game plan now if that should happen. At such times all communication between your family and your doctors and nurses may be done remotely—by phone or video—so it is critical that all staff know who you and your family have chosen as the spokesperson.

6. **Divide and conquer: organize your support system to help you both inside and outside of the hospital.**

- Everyone in your support system most likely has different strengths and availability to take on different tasks in caring for you.

- Often hospitals are far away from home, making it even more necessary to organize a "team" of caregivers who can share responsibilities across the home and hospital continuum.

- Decide who can step in for you on the home front and help care for children, pets, plants; make meals; and help out with essential chores.

- Decide if you need someone to help with your finances and personal bills, insurance, and hospital billing.
- When you are in the hospital, stagger visits so you will always have someone with you at **key moments** when mistakes and miscommunications can happen: the first night after surgery, medication times, mealtimes, doctors' rounds, treatment times, and most especially, staff shift changes (known as handoffs).
- Stagger visits so both you and your core support team of family and friends can get some rest.
- Stagger visits so you do not drive your roommate crazy—every patient desperately needs peace and quiet.
- Decide how much information you want to share about your illness or injury and with whom, and let your family know your wishes. Do you want someone to post updates on social media? Or do you want to start a CaringBridge.org site, which is specific to your health journey and has privacy protections?
- Decide how you want to stay connected to your family— by phone, Facetime, meeting apps—and make a plan.
- Fill out the My Important Health Information sheet at the end of Checklist 1 and give it to your medical team so they have your critical health and contact information.

7. Make sure your surgeon or hospital-based care team knows every prescription, over-the-counter medication, vitamin, and herbal remedy you take—and the dosages.

- It is very likely that your medications might change— sometimes radically—during a hospital stay. It is critical that your hospital team knows everything you are currently taking.

- The easiest thing to do is to brown-bag all of your medications and bring everything to your consultation prior to surgery (or take them with you to the emergency room). Just don't lose them! Give your meds to a family member to take home.
- Medical staff can read the labels for themselves and do not have to rely on your memory alone.
- You may have prescriptions from several different specialists for different conditions, which is why it is so important for your hospital health-care team to eyeball every single prescription to make sure there are no contraindications.
- Over-the-counter medications like aspirin or antihistamines as well as supplements such as herbs and vitamins can also interact with prescribed medications, which is another reason your hospital physicians need to know everything you are taking.
- **Alert your health-care team to allergies you might have to any medications.**
- There are a few excellent medication tracking apps listed in the Resources section.

8. Make sure your hospital care team knows whether you rely on sensory aids like glasses, hearing aids, and dentures. Also alert them to any medical implants in your body.

9. If possible, schedule surgery early in the day and early in the week.
- Common sense dictates that you want your surgical team to be rested and at the top of their game! Unless it's an emergency, why be wheeled into the operating

room after your surgeon has just completed two four-hour procedures back-to-back?

- The earlier to surgery, the earlier to recovery. Your status can be assessed during fully staffed hospital hours. Night and weekend shifts tend to be skeleton crews and, statistically, more medical errors occur at these times because of fatigue and understaffing. Also, doctors are simply less easy to contact at night and on weekends.

10. Find out all the details of your surgery, procedure, or treatment and expected recovery time. Take someone with you to all presurgery appointments to help listen and take notes. Ask if you can record the meeting. Here is important information to know to prepare for your hospital stay.

- First, ask your doctor to explain everything to you in plain language.
- Visual aids like a model or drawing can help explain surgical procedures.

Examples of questions to ask:
- What are the goals of this surgical procedure or treatment?
- What are the risks? Benefits? Alternatives?
- What will it cost? Who is coordinating with insurance?
- How long will the surgery/treatment last?
- How long will you be in the recovery room?
- When will your surgeon see you and your family after surgery? (Make sure the surgeon has contact information for your spokesperson and proxy!)

11. Get phone and pager numbers and email contacts for your doctors and any of their important support staff who may also be communicating with you and your family. Add this information to Checklist 9.

- How can you plan your discharge—especially if you will be going home the same day as your procedure? If you are not going home the same day, when is your anticipated discharge?
- If you are having outpatient surgery, can prescriptions be called in and picked up prior to the procedure? Can they be filled at the hospital pharmacy by a family member during your surgery?
- Are there typical reactions and side effects to the surgery, anesthesia, treatment, or medications that you might experience? What would be a bad reaction?
- How can you expect to feel in the first few hours? First few days?
- When will you know the actual outcome of the surgery/ treatment and whether it is successful? Right away? In a few days, weeks, or longer?
- When will you be "back to normal"?

12. What is the plan for surgical or treatment site management—how can you expect to heal and what type of aftercare is involved?

- Will you need to have a catheter, IV, drain, port, or any other invasive medical device? If so, how long will the device need to stay in and how will it be monitored?
- Be aware that any break in the skin barrier is a potential site for infection.
- What are the signs of infection or blockage for any invasive device so you can look out for it?
- Will you be discharged with any drains, ports, and so on still in place that you will need proper training to take care of?

13. What is the plan for pain management if you need it?
- Make sure you are clear on the type and dose of any pain medication and how and when it will be given to you during all phases of your hospital stay.
- What is the plan to assess pain management if a change is needed?

14. Will you need any blood transfusions? If so, can a compatible family member donate blood earmarked just for you?

15. Decide who will be with you the first night or two after surgery. Do not be alone! With sicker patients and fewer nurses, it is too easy to be overlooked. If family cannot be with you, you may want to look into having a private-duty nurse or nurse's aide stay with you, which the hospital can arrange although this is an out-of-pocket expense.

16. Can you readily access your complete electronic medical record (EMR), including lab, treatment, medications, and surgical reports, through the hospital's patient portal?
- It is important for you to have an organized file of your medical history in case you need additional medical treatment in the future, you move, or you change hospitals.
- Request hard copies now if a complete record is not easily accessible through the patient portal.
- You will need this documentation in case there are billing or insurance discrepancies or disputes over unexpected charges or reimbursements.

- These checklists provide a real-time, plain language documentation of your hospital stay and consequently provide an important reference point for all records and billings provided by the hospital.

HOSPITAL SPOTLIGHT

Don't Leave the Patient Alone the First Night . . . Ever

Marcy G. broke her wrist while tubing with her young sons. The break was so bad that she needed pins for her wrist. Unexpected delays at the hospital meant that her surgery started much later than expected. They had planned for morning surgery while her kids were in school so that her husband could pick them up at the end of the day. But that didn't happen and they didn't have a contingency plan. Her husband was assured once surgery was over and Marcy was in recovery that all went well and he should leave and go pick up the kids from a friend who had taken them home to her house. The anesthetic block would last all night, no worries. And they would get her pain meds going ASAP. After several hours in the recovery room, Marcy was wheeled into her hospital room just as the anesthetic block was starting to wear off. It was past midnight. Her nurse realized there was no call button at bedside and told Marcy she would be right back with a working call button and her pain meds. The nurse never came back. Marcy spent the night in agony, immobilized in a cast. No one heard her crying out. Finally, at 5 a.m. a resident came to check on her. Marcy's pain at that point was so severe she had to be put on a morphine drip for twenty-four hours, which also extended her hospital stay by two days.

My Important Health Information

Name: _____

DOB: _____

Insurance (name of carrier and member ID):

_____

My Important Contacts

Contact 1: _____

Phone: _____

Relationship to me: _____

Contact 2: _____

Phone: _____

Relationship to me: _____

My Health-Care Proxy: _____

Phone: _____

I have a health-care proxy: YES   NO   (see form attached)

I have a living will: YES   NO   (see form attached)

I use hearing aids ☐, glasses ☐, dentures ☐,
reading glasses ☐.

My current health conditions (including any implants):

_____

_____

Current list of medications, allergies to medication, and over-the-counter meds that I take (name/dose/schedule):

_____

_____

_____

My current doctors (name/number/why I see them):

_____

_____

Notes

_____

_____

_____

_____

_____

_____

_____

_____

_____

_____

_____

_____

_____

_____

_____

_____

_____

_____

_____

What to Bring

"If I were to give patients a very critical piece of advice—if you're coming to the hospital bring a family member. You know, you gotta bring someone who will sit with you and go get your Demerol for you, and help you if you fall in the bathroom, because that nurse is giving out meds and she's got ten patients and she's got IV lines."

—Anonymous Doctor, *New York Magazine*, June 18, 2007

Peak noise levels in hospitals can be as high as 85–90 dB, which is comparable to standing on a busy city street with traffic passing by.

Healthdesign.org

According to the 2018 Centers for Disease Control and Prevention's *National and State Healthcare-Associated Infections Progress Report*, each day, approximately one in thirty-one U.S. patients has at least one infection associated with his or her hospital care.

☐ **1.** Bring a family member or friend who can stay by your side.

☐ **2.** Have the following items on your person when you go to admitting or the ER:
- Photo ID.
- Insurance card or printout of front and back of card.
- A completed copy of the Important Health Information sheet (page 24) from Before You Go.
- Your phone and charger, along with a portable charger (fully charged) with cables because you may not be near an outlet or able to reach one. Make sure your phone has all of your important contact numbers. Your phone may be your primary source of communication with your family if the hospital has instituted a strict isolation policy with only virtual visits. Download playlists, eBooks, audio books, podcasts, games, and so on ahead of time.
- Your health-care proxy form and any other advance directives.
- Any sensory aids that you need (glasses, hearing aids with extra batteries, dentures, reading glasses) and their cases—all must be labeled with your name. Keep close track of these! After phones, hearing aids, glasses, and dentures are the items most often lost during a hospital stay. Losing anything that you depend on—to see, to hear, to eat—can seriously impair your recovery. Remember reading glasses if you need them.

In Your Hospital Go Bag

☐ **3.** This book and a few pens.

☐ **4.** An economy-size bottle of hand sanitizer, hand wipes, and disinfectant wipes for all the hard surfaces around your bed.

☐ **5.** Ear buds and/or headphones, ear plugs, and a sleep mask.
- Hospitals are noisy places! You might hear constant bleeps, beeps, blips from various machines and monitors by your bed; the loudspeaker above your bed; carts in the hallway; people in the hallway; your roommate's loud TV. Listening to relaxing music or wearing ear plugs can help you get some needed sleep.
- Hospitals are bright places! The lights are never off in a hospital and sleep is essential to a good outcome.

☐ **6.** Extra socks, a robe or a sweater, pajama bottoms if you can wear them.
- Hospitals are cold places! Your circulation is already going to be compromised by being confined to a bed and most hospitals have intense air-conditioning. Being cold can suppress the immune system and slow down healing!
- The hospital will give you grip socks to walk in to help prevent falls. But never get back into bed with socks you have used for walking—change them to avoid spreading germs to your sheets.

☐ **7.** Toiletries, especially facial wipes and mouthwash.
- The hospital will provide a small kit with a toothbrush, toothpaste, comb, and so on, but you might want to bring your own supplies from home.

- You might not be able to get out of bed to brush your teeth and wash your face—let alone shower—or you just might not be up to it. A swish of mouthwash and a facial wipe can be refreshing.

8. **Tablet and/or laptop with chargers if you need them but no other items of value like your wallet or jewelry.**
   - These electronic devices can easily get lost or stolen, but they have become central to how we live our lives, work, entertain ourselves, and stay connected.
   - We may be moving into a new hospital landscape where virtual communication with your family will be more of a norm if visitation rules become more restricted. Think about apps to facilitate family "meetings."
   - To keep them safe, label them and always put your phone and other devices in the room safe before you go to sleep or if you are leaving your room for any reason—even to walk the halls.
   - Hospitals are not responsible for any personal belongings that are lost.

9. **Books, crosswords, Sudoku, and so on if you prefer print copies. Hospitals actually use challenging games to help maintain cognitive health for bedbound patients.**

10. **A photograph that reminds you of your life outside the hospital.**

Have a Plan to Combat Hospital Chaos So You Don't Lose Your Mind

Catherine was hospitalized on bed rest for the last two weeks of her third pregnancy. She had the dreaded bed by the door . . . right outside the nurses' station. Her roommate, another woman on bed rest, would have six or seven family visitors all day every day. Catherine was able to ignore it with a good pair of noise-canceling headphones, her tablet, and her streaming subscriptions. She tuned out everything by working through the movies on her never-had-a-chance-to-see list. At night she drifted off to sleep listening to music and wearing a sleep mask.

Notes

_____

_____

_____

_____

_____

_____

_____

_____

_____

_____

_____

_____

_____

_____

_____

_____

_____

_____

_____

During Your Stay

"Doctors desperately need patients and their families and friends to help them think. Without their help, physicians are denied key clues to what is really wrong....Language is still the bedrock of clinical practice."

—Dr. Jerome Groopman, *How Doctors Think*

A recent study found that as many as 75 percent
of patients can't name any doctor who took care
of them in the hospital.

> "Fewer Doctors Visit Their Patients in the
> Hospital," *AARP Bulletin Today*

U.S. nurses consistently report that hospital
nurse staffing levels are inadequate to provide
safe and effective care.

> The Aiken Study, *Journal of the American
> Medical Association* 288, no. 16 (October
> 2002): 1987–1993

☐ **1. Make names and contact numbers a must in all hospital interactions. Get to know your nurses and aides. Get the number for the nurses, station for your floor or unit.**

- Names are the first thing to go in a hospital setting but the most important in encouraging a human connection in the hospital.
- Nurses are the human face of technology-driven care. They can be powerful allies for you. Nurses best know your daily care plan.
- Hospital aides help you with important basic needs like bathing, toileting, dressing, and feeding. They help you reposition in bed or move from bed to chair or wheelchair as needed. They also take your temperature and vital signs. They do not administer medications but can alert your nurses to any medication needs. Of all your hospital care team, aides will be the staff you see most and really get to know.
- Each hospital has a different nurse/patient ratio as well as aide/patient ratio, but your nurses and aides can always use more help. Family provides much, if not most, of day-to-day comfort care.
- Find out if you will have a hospitalist supervising and coordinating all your hospital care. This will be a new but important doctor for you. As care grows more complex and multiple surgeons and specialists may be involved the hospitalist is the physician as quarterback. He or she works specifically for the hospital, as opposed to a private practice, and specializes in managing the complexities of daily high-tech intensive care.
- Get the names, cell, pager, and email information for all key members of you hospital care team—this can

include your surgeon, specialist doctors, hospitalist, key residents, social worker or case manager, nurse manager for your unit, the nurses' station phone number, and any physician assistants or nurse practitioners who work with any of your specialists and add them to Checklist 9.

2. **Consider your hospital room your temporary home— learn how everything works.**

- Find out how to work the TV, the phone, the bed, and especially the call button. Make sure that everything works.

- Climate control is essential to your comfort—and ability to heal. Make sure you have enough blankets and pillows to keep warm and comfortable.

- Real estate is everything in a hospital. A bed by the window or a quieter room can make a world of difference to a patient and help or hinder recovery. If you are uncomfortable with your bed, room, or roommate, it is okay to ask for a change.

- Your bedside table is command central. Keep your phone and any other electronic devices, chargers, earbuds, and headphones within reach (but put them in the room safe when you leave your room). Never leave them in or on your bed when you are out of it—or they might wind up in the hospital laundry!

- Store your glasses, hearing aids, or dentures with their labeled cases in the top drawer for safekeeping when you are not using them.

- Keep earplugs and a sleep mask handy.

- Put your economy-size hand sanitizer within easy reach for you. All hospital rooms have a wall dispenser of hand sanitizer but you may not be able to get out of

During Your Stay

bed. Also it is one more visual reminder of how important hand hygiene is—for everyone including you.

- Keep pens and this book handy to jot down notes and reminders.
- Keep your playlists, books, Sudoku, and crosswords handy. Playing challenging games can maintain cognitive health in an environment set up to be disorienting.

☐ **3. Make room cleanliness an absolute priority.**
- Think of all the people who move in and out of a hospital room. Hospital rooms are really dirty—period. Three-quarters of patients' rooms are contaminated with bacteria that can cause staph infections.
- Family should use antibacterial wipes to clean high-contact or often touched surfaces—tabletops and drawer pulls, chair armrests, bed railings, the call button, the TV remote, doorknobs, bathroom fixtures, and any personal electronic devices you have brought. Wiping down surfaces should be done several times a day by family. Always wear latex gloves and wash your hands afterward. There are glove dispensers in every room. There are also multiple dispensers of antibacterial wipes on every hospital floor if you have not brought your own or run out.

☐ **4. Wash your hands frequently and use a hand sanitizer whenever and wherever one is available.**
- Patients are constantly exposed to surface contaminants on items around them that hospital staff touch throughout the day while providing care: bed rails, food trays, IV poles, call buttons, and many more. You need to wash your hands or use hand sanitizer as often as anyone else.

- Lapses in hand hygiene are the number one cause of hospital-acquired infections. Ask all health-care staff to wash their hands before touching you. Don't be shy about this.

5. Make the whiteboard in your room the information bulletin board and communication command center and let your care team know.

- The whiteboard lets you know the day, date, and what nurses and aides are on duty and what their shifts are. You and your family will know who is on duty for you for each 24-hour cycle.
- Most importantly, their schedules will let you know when the handoff is—when they change shifts. Statistically, these are the times when miscommunications between care team members happen most frequently and medical errors can happen. Always compare your own "status" notes with your nurses when they begin their rounds so you can make sure everyone is on the same page.
- Remember "you" addresses collective you—so adapt accordingly in terms of who can add this information— most patients may not be capable. Add important contact information for you: your primary family bedside advocate for the day (in case that person is getting a coffee when the doctor comes by—you want to alert them to come back), your health-care proxy, your family spokesperson.
- These family contacts are especially important if your family is restricted from visiting you for any reason. Ask your nurse to make a note on your whiteboard for doctors to call your family contact when they round to include them in any bedside meetings.

- Make a visible note on the whiteboard if you need an interpreter. All hospitals have to supply interpreters— either in person or via phone or video.
- Make a note if you wear hearing aids, glasses, or dentures. This is vital patient information.
- You can also use the whiteboard as a reminder for important questions you might want to ask your doctors when they round. Write it down on the board so both you and your care team can see it.
- Ask your nurses when your doctors typically round every day and add it to the whiteboard so your family will know their daily schedule and can be there with you.

6. **Stay hydrated and nourished.**
   - Staying hydrated, having enough fluids, is key to recovery.
   - Sucking on ice chips can be a good alternative if you are unable or don't want to drink fluids.
   - Hospital food is the worst kind of institutional, low-fiber food. It, along with being bedbound, can contribute to constipation, which can usher in its own host of problems.
   - Ask your doctors if it is okay to bring in simple, fiber-rich food as well as to take a daily probiotic.

7. **Start preparing for discharge from the first day of your hospital stay.**
   - As soon as possible, ask to meet with the social worker or case manager on your care team if that is the person who will be your discharge planner. If not, ask your nurse who is handling discharge for you.
   - See Checklist 7 for the discharge planning checklist.

8. Set up your Patient Portal.
- Have your nurse or case manager help you set up your patient portal if you have not already done so. Include a family member if you give them permission to access your protected health information for practical caregiving needs.
- Make sure that all lab work, films, and medical orders are accessible to you through the portal or ask for hard copies now.

9. Hold a hand.
- Patients in hospitals are touched-deprived. Touch is consoling and healing.

10. Consider whether a visit from your pastor, priest, minister, Rabbi, Imam, Guru, Buddhist priest, or any other spiritual advisor will offer you solace, support, or guidance.

11. Express thanks to your doctors, nurses, aides, and other support staff for their help in caring for you.

12. Keep connected to your family and friends.

13. Explore complementary care offerings if you are interested. Many hospitals offer healing modalities like Reiki, breath work, light-touch massage, acupuncture, and hypnosis. Some hospitals also offer pet therapy.

14. Find moments for love and laughter.
- Family and friends are the primary providers of comfort care during any hospital stay. You know the patient best and what little things mean a lot to them. Try to weave reminders of the life before a hospital stay into

During Your Stay

your time with the patient—to comfort them and to counter the alien environment they find themselves in.

- Laughing releases the body's natural painkiller—endorphins.

15. Maintain Checklists 4–6. These three checklists work together to monitor and manage your daily care and to help you effectively partner with your care team.

Notes

Master Medication List

"Physical examination and history-taking are still the origins of diagnosis, but seem not as important as they were only thirty years ago....The ultimate mainstay of diagnosis is not data, information, or even knowledge—it is judgment."

—Sherwin Nuland, *The Soul of Medicine*

Pain was associated with the greatest objective sleep loss, highlighting the need for proactive screening and management of patient pain to improve sleep in hospitals.

American Academy of Sleep Medicine 13, no. 2 (2017): 301–306

Medication errors injure 1.5 million people per year.

Journal of Community Hospital Internal Medicine Perspectives 6, no. 4 (2016)

☐ **1.** Review each hospital medication carefully with each prescribing doctor as well as your nurse. Why do you need it? What is the dosage and schedule? Do you need to ask for a medication as with most pain medication or is it dispensed on a regular schedule?

☐ **2.** Note if there are any changes from your regular, pre-hospitalization prescription regimen. If there are any changes or omissions, ask for a medication review with your hospitalist or whichever doctor is in charge of overall care and ask why. Sometimes it is an error that one of your medications is left off the hospital list.

☐ **3.** Adapt the master medication list as needed to reflect your own individual hospital medication plan.

☐ **4.** Fill out information boxes for each medication in clear, legible handwriting.

☐ **5.** Checklists 4 and 5 work hand in hand.
- Checklist 4 is your master medication list for the entire time that you are in the hospital. It is your medication manager by providing a complete record of every medication along with its start and end dates.
- Checklist 5, the Daily Medication Log, is how you monitor that each and every medication given to you—on a daily basis—is the right drug and dosage for you and arrives on time.
- Both can help you be vigilant about *polypharmacy*. Polypharmacy is when you take a lot of medications for various medical conditions that are prescribed by

many different doctors. It creates an opportunity for bad interactions. Checklist 4 lets you see the whole list. Checklist 5 keeps you alert for side effects.

Follow the guide for filling out the boxes:

- DRUG NAME: Write down the name of the medication—even if it is long and incomprehensible—and even though you will probably rely on what each medication actually looks like to self-monitor on a daily basis.
- DESCRIPTION: The description box (small blue pill, big white capsule, etc.) is the visual reference, which is the easiest way to check each medication dispensed to you. Then write down the route or method of how it is administered in this box—for example, if meds are injections, IVs, puffs on an inhaler, or suppositories.
- WHY: Keep it simple and concise—"heart med," "blood pressure," "nausea." It is important to understand the "why" of every medication going into your body.
- DOCTOR: Write down the name of the doctor who prescribed each medication. With the potential for multiple specialists, this will help you keep track of who is prescribing what—and why. Make sure you review this complete medication list with each prescribing doctor so no contraindications are overlooked.
- DAILY SCHEDULE—TIME/DOSAGE: Dosage and schedule go hand in hand. Medication amounts can vary over the course of the day—you may get 5 mg of something in the morning and 10 mg at night. Medications are normally administered on a regular schedule. What is yours? By knowing your meds, their dosage, and schedule you can actively guard against medication errors.

- SPECIAL INSTRUCTIONS: Make a note here if a medication should be taken with food, on an empty stomach, only as needed, and so on.
- ADVERSE REACTIONS: This box is for any bad reactions or side effects that *you*, the individual patient, might be feeling. Make sure you understand possible side effects for each medication. A brief description, like "dry mouth" or "dizziness," helps you track side effects. Tell your doctors and nurses!
- START AND END DATES: Track start and end dates for each medication. This box is important for a number of reasons. It clearly indicates how long you have been taking something. It is also a useful record to check charges on your hospital bill and insurance claims.

Medical Abbreviations

These are just some of the most common abbreviations for your reference. Ask your doctor or nurse to explain abbreviations for your medications.

Abbreviation	Meaning
Ac	before meals
bid	twice a day
gt	drop
hs	at bedtime
po	by mouth
pc	after meals
prn	as needed
q3h	every three hours
qd	every day
qid	four times a day
tid	three times a day

Know Your Medication Schedule

My brother-in-law Steven had complex open-heart surgery in an attempt to remove a cardiac sarcoma—a rare cancerous tumor. When he was moved from the ICU to a regular hospital room, there was a mix-up in communication with our family—we thought he was supposed to get pain medication every four hours on a strict schedule. By the time the fourth hour was approaching, Steven was in agony. He asked me to go check with his nurse that his pain medication was on its way. I ran to find his nurse, who looked up his chart and said, "Oh, he can have pain medication every *three* hours but he has to ask for it." No one gave us these instructions. I told her it had been four hours since his last pain medication and he was suffering terribly. His nurse brought him his pain medication right away, but it took him that much longer to get his pain under control. No one had come in to check on him for a few hours and we were all under the misconception that his pain medication was on a specific schedule and we were supposed to just wait for it. We had fallen into the passive patient trap.

Master Medication List

DRUG NAME	DESCRIPTION	DAILY SCHEDULE *2X*	
Lasix	*white oval tablet*	TIME	DOSAGE
DOCTOR	WHY	*8 am*	*4 mg*
Smith	*water retention*	*5 pm*	*4 mg*
SPECIAL INSTRUCTIONS			
ADVERSE REACTIONS			
DATE STARTED			
DATE ENDED	*10/6/2010*		

DRUG NAME	DESCRIPTION	DAILY SCHEDULE *1X*	
Glipizide XL	*small, round white tablet*	TIME	DOSAGE
DOCTOR	WHY	*8 am*	*5 mg*
Smith	*diabetes*		
SPECIAL INSTRUCTIONS	*with breakfast*		
ADVERSE REACTIONS			
DATE STARTED	*10/5/2010*		
DATE ENDED			

DRUG NAME	DESCRIPTION	DAILY SCHEDULE *1X*	
insulin	*shot*	TIME	DOSAGE
DOCTOR	WHY	*8 am*	*10 mg*
Smith	*diabetes*	*12 pm*	*10 mg*
SPECIAL INSTRUCTIONS	*15 mins. before meals*	*5 pm*	*10 mg*
ADVERSE REACTIONS			
DATE STARTED	*10/5/2010*		
DATE ENDED			

SAMPLE

Master Medication List

DRUG NAME	DESCRIPTION	DAILY SCHEDULE	
		TIME	DOSAGE
DOCTOR	WHY		
SPECIAL INSTRUCTIONS			
ADVERSE REACTIONS			
DATE STARTED			
DATE ENDED			

DRUG NAME	DESCRIPTION	DAILY SCHEDULE	
		TIME	DOSAGE
DOCTOR	WHY		
SPECIAL INSTRUCTIONS			
ADVERSE REACTIONS			
DATE STARTED			
DATE ENDED			

DRUG NAME	DESCRIPTION	DAILY SCHEDULE	
		TIME	DOSAGE
DOCTOR	WHY		
SPECIAL INSTRUCTIONS			
ADVERSE REACTIONS			
DATE STARTED			
DATE ENDED			

DRUG NAME	DESCRIPTION	DAILY SCHEDULE	
		TIME	DOSAGE
DOCTOR	WHY		
SPECIAL INSTRUCTIONS			
ADVERSE REACTIONS			
DATE STARTED			
DATE ENDED			

DRUG NAME	DESCRIPTION	DAILY SCHEDULE	
		TIME	DOSAGE
DOCTOR	WHY		
SPECIAL INSTRUCTIONS			
ADVERSE REACTIONS			
DATE STARTED			
DATE ENDED			

DRUG NAME	DESCRIPTION	DAILY SCHEDULE	
		TIME	DOSAGE
DOCTOR	WHY		
SPECIAL INSTRUCTIONS			
ADVERSE REACTIONS			
DATE STARTED			
DATE ENDED			

Master Medication List

DRUG NAME	DESCRIPTION	DAILY SCHEDULE	
		TIME	DOSAGE
DOCTOR	WHY		
SPECIAL INSTRUCTIONS			
ADVERSE REACTIONS			
DATE STARTED			
DATE ENDED			

DRUG NAME	DESCRIPTION	DAILY SCHEDULE	
		TIME	DOSAGE
DOCTOR	WHY		
SPECIAL INSTRUCTIONS			
ADVERSE REACTIONS			
DATE STARTED			
DATE ENDED			

DRUG NAME	DESCRIPTION	DAILY SCHEDULE	
		TIME	DOSAGE
DOCTOR	WHY		
SPECIAL INSTRUCTIONS			
ADVERSE REACTIONS			
DATE STARTED			
DATE ENDED			

DRUG NAME	DESCRIPTION	DAILY SCHEDULE	
		TIME	DOSAGE
DOCTOR	WHY		
SPECIAL INSTRUCTIONS			
ADVERSE REACTIONS			
DATE STARTED			
DATE ENDED			

DRUG NAME	DESCRIPTION	DAILY SCHEDULE	
		TIME	DOSAGE
DOCTOR	WHY		
SPECIAL INSTRUCTIONS			
ADVERSE REACTIONS			
DATE STARTED			
DATE ENDED			

DRUG NAME	DESCRIPTION	DAILY SCHEDULE	
		TIME	DOSAGE
DOCTOR	WHY		
SPECIAL INSTRUCTIONS			
ADVERSE REACTIONS			
DATE STARTED			
DATE ENDED			

Master Medication List

DRUG NAME	DESCRIPTION	DAILY SCHEDULE	
		TIME	DOSAGE
DOCTOR	WHY		
SPECIAL INSTRUCTIONS			
ADVERSE REACTIONS			
DATE STARTED			
DATE ENDED			

DRUG NAME	DESCRIPTION	DAILY SCHEDULE	
		TIME	DOSAGE
DOCTOR	WHY		
SPECIAL INSTRUCTIONS			
ADVERSE REACTIONS			
DATE STARTED			
DATE ENDED			

DRUG NAME	DESCRIPTION	DAILY SCHEDULE	
		TIME	DOSAGE
DOCTOR	WHY		
SPECIAL INSTRUCTIONS			
ADVERSE REACTIONS			
DATE STARTED			
DATE ENDED			

DRUG NAME	DESCRIPTION	DAILY SCHEDULE	
		TIME	DOSAGE
DOCTOR	WHY		
SPECIAL INSTRUCTIONS			
ADVERSE REACTIONS			
DATE STARTED			
DATE ENDED			

DRUG NAME	DESCRIPTION	DAILY SCHEDULE	
		TIME	DOSAGE
DOCTOR	WHY		
SPECIAL INSTRUCTIONS			
ADVERSE REACTIONS			
DATE STARTED			
DATE ENDED			

DRUG NAME	DESCRIPTION	DAILY SCHEDULE	
		TIME	DOSAGE
DOCTOR	WHY		
SPECIAL INSTRUCTIONS			
ADVERSE REACTIONS			
DATE STARTED			
DATE ENDED			

Master Medication List

DRUG NAME	DESCRIPTION	DAILY SCHEDULE	
		TIME	DOSAGE
DOCTOR	WHY		
SPECIAL INSTRUCTIONS			
ADVERSE REACTIONS			
DATE STARTED			
DATE ENDED			

DRUG NAME	DESCRIPTION	DAILY SCHEDULE	
		TIME	DOSAGE
DOCTOR	WHY		
SPECIAL INSTRUCTIONS			
ADVERSE REACTIONS			
DATE STARTED			
DATE ENDED			

DRUG NAME	DESCRIPTION	DAILY SCHEDULE	
		TIME	DOSAGE
DOCTOR	WHY		
SPECIAL INSTRUCTIONS			
ADVERSE REACTIONS			
DATE STARTED			
DATE ENDED			

Master Medication List

DRUG NAME	DESCRIPTION	DAILY SCHEDULE	
		TIME	DOSAGE
DOCTOR	WHY		
SPECIAL INSTRUCTIONS			
ADVERSE REACTIONS			
DATE STARTED			
DATE ENDED			

DRUG NAME	DESCRIPTION	DAILY SCHEDULE	
		TIME	DOSAGE
DOCTOR	WHY		
SPECIAL INSTRUCTIONS			
ADVERSE REACTIONS			
DATE STARTED			
DATE ENDED			

DRUG NAME	DESCRIPTION	DAILY SCHEDULE	
		TIME	DOSAGE
DOCTOR	WHY		
SPECIAL INSTRUCTIONS			
ADVERSE REACTIONS			
DATE STARTED			
DATE ENDED			

Master Medication List

Daily Medication Log

"The young physician starts life with twenty drugs for each disease, and the old physician ends life with one drug for twenty diseases."

—Sir William Osler

More medication errors occur on the night shift.

Johns Hopkins Nursing, April 7, 2017

About 75 percent of medication errors are attributed to a distraction.

National Center for Biotechnology
Information: Medication Errors,
February 18, 2020

The Five Rights for Safe Medication

This is the simplest, most efficient checklist taught to all nurses.
Use it to review each and every time a medication is given to you:

☐ **1.** The Right Drug

☐ **2.** The Right Dose

☐ **3.** The Right Route (i.e., method: injection, oral, topical ointment, inhalant, etc.)

☐ **4.** The Right Schedule

☐ **5.** The Right Patient

Daily Medication Log

DATE:	10.6.2010		DAY:	#5 in hospital	

TIME	DRUG	DOSAGE	ROUTE		ON TIME?
8 AM	Lasix	4 mg.	☑ ORAL ☐ IV ☐ SHOT ☐ OTHER		☑
8 A	Glipizide	5 mg.	☑ ORAL ☐ IV ☐ SHOT ☐ OTHER		☑
8 A	Insulin	10 units	☐ ORAL ☐ IV ☑ SHOT ☐ OTHER		☑
8 A	Seroquel	50 mg.	☑ ORAL ☐ IV ☐ SHOT ☐ OTHER		☐
8 A	Depakote	250 mg.	☑ ORAL ☐ IV ☐ SHOT ☐ OTHER		☐
12 P	Insulin	10 units	☐ ORAL ☐ IV ☑ SHOT ☐ OTHER		☐
5 P	Lasix	4 mg.	☑ ORAL ☐ IV ☐ SHOT ☐ OTHER		☐
5 P	Glipizide XL	5 mg.	☑ ORAL ☐ IV ☐ SHOT ☐ OTHER		☐
5 P	Insulin	10 units	☑ ORAL ☐ IV ☐ SHOT ☐ OTHER		☐

NOTES:

SAMPLE

DATE: _____   **DAY:** _____

TIME	DRUG	DOSAGE	ROUTE	ON TIME?
			☐ ORAL ☐ IV ☐ SHOT ☐ OTHER	☐
			☐ ORAL ☐ IV ☐ SHOT ☐ OTHER	☐
			☐ ORAL ☐ IV ☐ SHOT ☐ OTHER	☐
			☐ ORAL ☐ IV ☐ SHOT ☐ OTHER	☐
			☐ ORAL ☐ IV ☐ SHOT ☐ OTHER	☐
			☐ ORAL ☐ IV ☐ SHOT ☐ OTHER	☐
			☐ ORAL ☐ IV ☐ SHOT ☐ OTHER	☐
			☐ ORAL ☐ IV ☐ SHOT ☐ OTHER	☐
			☐ ORAL ☐ IV ☐ SHOT ☐ OTHER	☐

NOTES:

Daily Medication Log

DATE: _____   **DAY:** _____

TIME	DRUG	DOSAGE	ROUTE				ON TIME?
			☐ ORAL	☐ IV	☐ SHOT	☐ OTHER	☐
			☐ ORAL	☐ IV	☐ SHOT	☐ OTHER	☐
			☐ ORAL	☐ IV	☐ SHOT	☐ OTHER	☐
			☐ ORAL	☐ IV	☐ SHOT	☐ OTHER	☐
			☐ ORAL	☐ IV	☐ SHOT	☐ OTHER	☐
			☐ ORAL	☐ IV	☐ SHOT	☐ OTHER	☐
			☐ ORAL	☐ IV	☐ SHOT	☐ OTHER	☐
			☐ ORAL	☐ IV	☐ SHOT	☐ OTHER	☐
			☐ ORAL	☐ IV	☐ SHOT	☐ OTHER	☐

NOTES:

DATE: _____   **DAY:** _____

TIME	DRUG	DOSAGE	ROUTE	ON TIME?
			☐ ORAL ☐ IV ☐ SHOT ☐ OTHER	☐
			☐ ORAL ☐ IV ☐ SHOT ☐ OTHER	☐
			☐ ORAL ☐ IV ☐ SHOT ☐ OTHER	☐
			☐ ORAL ☐ IV ☐ SHOT ☐ OTHER	☐
			☐ ORAL ☐ IV ☐ SHOT ☐ OTHER	☐
			☐ ORAL ☐ IV ☐ SHOT ☐ OTHER	☐
			☐ ORAL ☐ IV ☐ SHOT ☐ OTHER	☐
			☐ ORAL ☐ IV ☐ SHOT ☐ OTHER	☐
			☐ ORAL ☐ IV ☐ SHOT ☐ OTHER	☐

NOTES:

DATE: _____   **DAY:** _____

TIME	DRUG	DOSAGE	ROUTE				ON TIME?
			☐ ORAL	☐ IV	☐ SHOT	☐ OTHER	☐
			☐ ORAL	☐ IV	☐ SHOT	☐ OTHER	☐
			☐ ORAL	☐ IV	☐ SHOT	☐ OTHER	☐
			☐ ORAL	☐ IV	☐ SHOT	☐ OTHER	☐
			☐ ORAL	☐ IV	☐ SHOT	☐ OTHER	☐
			☐ ORAL	☐ IV	☐ SHOT	☐ OTHER	☐
			☐ ORAL	☐ IV	☐ SHOT	☐ OTHER	☐
			☐ ORAL	☐ IV	☐ SHOT	☐ OTHER	☐
			☐ ORAL	☐ IV	☐ SHOT	☐ OTHER	☐

NOTES:

DATE: _____   **DAY:** _____

TIME	DRUG	DOSAGE	ROUTE	ON TIME?
			☐ ORAL ☐ IV ☐ SHOT ☐ OTHER	☐
			☐ ORAL ☐ IV ☐ SHOT ☐ OTHER	☐
			☐ ORAL ☐ IV ☐ SHOT ☐ OTHER	☐
			☐ ORAL ☐ IV ☐ SHOT ☐ OTHER	☐
			☐ ORAL ☐ IV ☐ SHOT ☐ OTHER	☐
			☐ ORAL ☐ IV ☐ SHOT ☐ OTHER	☐
			☐ ORAL ☐ IV ☐ SHOT ☐ OTHER	☐
			☐ ORAL ☐ IV ☐ SHOT ☐ OTHER	☐
			☐ ORAL ☐ IV ☐ SHOT ☐ OTHER	☐

NOTES:

DATE: _____   **DAY:** _____

TIME	DRUG	DOSAGE	ROUTE				ON TIME?
			☐ ORAL	☐ IV	☐ SHOT	☐ OTHER	☐
			☐ ORAL	☐ IV	☐ SHOT	☐ OTHER	☐
			☐ ORAL	☐ IV	☐ SHOT	☐ OTHER	☐
			☐ ORAL	☐ IV	☐ SHOT	☐ OTHER	☐
			☐ ORAL	☐ IV	☐ SHOT	☐ OTHER	☐
			☐ ORAL	☐ IV	☐ SHOT	☐ OTHER	☐
			☐ ORAL	☐ IV	☐ SHOT	☐ OTHER	☐
			☐ ORAL	☐ IV	☐ SHOT	☐ OTHER	☐
			☐ ORAL	☐ IV	☐ SHOT	☐ OTHER	☐

NOTES:

DATE: _____ **DAY:** _____

TIME	DRUG	DOSAGE	ROUTE				ON TIME?
			☐ ORAL	☐ IV	☐ SHOT	☐ OTHER	☐
			☐ ORAL	☐ IV	☐ SHOT	☐ OTHER	☐
			☐ ORAL	☐ IV	☐ SHOT	☐ OTHER	☐
			☐ ORAL	☐ IV	☐ SHOT	☐ OTHER	☐
			☐ ORAL	☐ IV	☐ SHOT	☐ OTHER	☐
			☐ ORAL	☐ IV	☐ SHOT	☐ OTHER	☐
			☐ ORAL	☐ IV	☐ SHOT	☐ OTHER	☐
			☐ ORAL	☐ IV	☐ SHOT	☐ OTHER	☐
			☐ ORAL	☐ IV	☐ SHOT	☐ OTHER	☐

NOTES:

Daily Medication Log

DATE: _____   **DAY:** _____

TIME	DRUG	DOSAGE	ROUTE	ON TIME?
			☐ ORAL ☐ IV ☐ SHOT ☐ OTHER	☐
			☐ ORAL ☐ IV ☐ SHOT ☐ OTHER	☐
			☐ ORAL ☐ IV ☐ SHOT ☐ OTHER	☐
			☐ ORAL ☐ IV ☐ SHOT ☐ OTHER	☐
			☐ ORAL ☐ IV ☐ SHOT ☐ OTHER	☐
			☐ ORAL ☐ IV ☐ SHOT ☐ OTHER	☐
			☐ ORAL ☐ IV ☐ SHOT ☐ OTHER	☐
			☐ ORAL ☐ IV ☐ SHOT ☐ OTHER	☐
			☐ ORAL ☐ IV ☐ SHOT ☐ OTHER	☐

NOTES:

DATE: _____ **DAY:** _____

TIME	DRUG	DOSAGE	ROUTE				ON TIME?
			☐ ORAL	☐ IV	☐ SHOT	☐ OTHER	☐
			☐ ORAL	☐ IV	☐ SHOT	☐ OTHER	☐
			☐ ORAL	☐ IV	☐ SHOT	☐ OTHER	☐
			☐ ORAL	☐ IV	☐ SHOT	☐ OTHER	☐
			☐ ORAL	☐ IV	☐ SHOT	☐ OTHER	☐
			☐ ORAL	☐ IV	☐ SHOT	☐ OTHER	☐
			☐ ORAL	☐ IV	☐ SHOT	☐ OTHER	☐
			☐ ORAL	☐ IV	☐ SHOT	☐ OTHER	☐
			☐ ORAL	☐ IV	☐ SHOT	☐ OTHER	☐

NOTES:

DATE: _____ **DAY:** _____

TIME	DRUG	DOSAGE	ROUTE	ON TIME?
			☐ ORAL ☐ IV ☐ SHOT ☐ OTHER	☐
			☐ ORAL ☐ IV ☐ SHOT ☐ OTHER	☐
			☐ ORAL ☐ IV ☐ SHOT ☐ OTHER	☐
			☐ ORAL ☐ IV ☐ SHOT ☐ OTHER	☐
			☐ ORAL ☐ IV ☐ SHOT ☐ OTHER	☐
			☐ ORAL ☐ IV ☐ SHOT ☐ OTHER	☐
			☐ ORAL ☐ IV ☐ SHOT ☐ OTHER	☐
			☐ ORAL ☐ IV ☐ SHOT ☐ OTHER	☐
			☐ ORAL ☐ IV ☐ SHOT ☐ OTHER	☐

NOTES:

Families Catch Medication Errors

Medication mistakes happen all the time in the hospital—usually because of distraction that results in a chart omission or a name mix-up or something of the kind. Consider what *nearly* happened to Katie with medication errors—all within a 24-hour period—only prevented by her family who were keeping vigil at her bedside. Katie was on Coumadin for a heart condition—a blood-thinning medication that is a extremely powerful, volatile drug. She was given her daily dose, but the nurse failed to make a note of it in Katie's chart. Two hours later, after a shift change, a new nurse came to dispense her daily dose of Coumadin, but Katie's family was there and stopped her. The nurse was insistent, but so was Katie's family. The error was discovered when a record from the hospital pharmacy was requested and checked—showing that indeed Coumadin had been ordered and delivered to her earlier. Later that night, Katie's nurse came to dispense her dose of methadone. Katie had never taken methadone in her life. Once again, her family stopped the nurse over the objections of the resident who prescribed it. Although he was annoyed, the resident double-checked his records and realized the methadone was meant for a patient on another floor with the same last name.

Daily Journal

"To hinder the description of illness...there is a poverty of language.... The merest schoolgirl, when she falls in love, has Shakespeare or Keats to speak her mind for her; but let a sufferer try to describe a pain in his head to a doctor and language at once runs dry."

—Virginia Woolf, *On Being Ill*

An estimated 70 percent of medical complications and deaths among hospitalized patients can be prevented if early signs of deterioration in clinical conditions are identified and followed by immediate assessment and appropriate intervention.

Critical Care Nurse 27, no. 1 (2007): 20–27

Hospital-induced delirium is common in ICU patients, affecting 60–80 percent of ventilated patients and 20–50 percent of nonventilated patients.

Critical Care Clinics 29, no. 1 (2013)

Daily Reminders

Use the following checklist as a starting point each day to help you (your collective "you" of family and friends) manage and monitor your care. Adapt it to your individual needs. It provides a template to capture a detailed day-to-day history of your hospital stay to create your own daily progress notes—the lay version of your medical chart.

☐ **1.** Who are your nurses and what are their shifts? When is the handoff (shift change)? Always have your family check in with the night nurse before her shift ends if you have been alone overnight. Is there any important information, either you or a family member should add to your Daily Journal notes for that day?

☐ **2.** Which doctor is supervising and coordinating your overall care today? Do you have a hospitalist? What is his/her shift? When do doctors round?

☐ **3.** Use the red flag box for important reminders if you sense something is wrong—like a reddened IV site, a strange reaction to a medication, too much pain, not going to the bathroom, and so on. Alert your nurses and doctors.

☐ **4.** Do you have any additional surgeries, treatments, physical therapy or occupational therapy sessions, or other tests happening today? Do you understand why you need this?

☐ **5.** Has there been any change in medication? Who ordered it and why?

6. How does the surgical site look and feel? When was it last checked and by whom?

7. Is any invasive or monitoring device (catheters, IV, ports, feeding tubes, ventilators) hooked up to you being checked regularly for signs of infection or blockages? Can it be removed today? Tomorrow?

8. Are you in pain? What does the pain feel like? Dull, achy, sharp, new, or unusual? Pain is a signal that something is wrong so tell your nurses and doctors if you are in discomfort.

9. How do you feel? Better, worse, hungry, anxious, restless? Are you able to get out of bed? Walk the halls? Can you go to the bathroom? Are you constipated?

10. If bedbound, are you being checked regularly for pressure sores? Are you being turned? Is an alternating pressure mattress being used to provide relief? If not, ask for one.

11. Ask whoever is at bedside with you to be on alert for these signs of hospital delirium: Do you seem yourself? Not sleeping at all or at odd times? Sleeping too much? Seem too quiet? Confused or disoriented? Bring this to the attention of your doctors and nurses. See the Hospital Delirium Fact Sheet.

12. Are you being transferred to the ICU from your medical or surgical floor? Do you and your family understand why? See the ICU Family Information Fact Sheet.

☐ **13.** Do you feel that you and your family might benefit from having a family meeting with your hospital care team? These are extremely helpful meetings when everyone can come together to discuss complex care—and get on the same page. Are there family conflicts about care goals? Confusion about information from different doctors? Concerns about reactions to drugs or therapy? Communication gaps? Ask your nurse how to organize this important family resource.

☐ **14.** Would a palliative care consult be helpful to you? If so, ask your nurse or doctor to arrange a consultation. Palliative care is about the whole person, not just the illness or injury. It is specialized medical care that focuses on symptom management (shortness of breath, fatigue, etc.), pain management, and improving overall quality of life for anyone facing a serious or chronic illness. Most hospitals have palliative care services. Palliative care can be especially helpful for pain management. See Resources for more information about palliative care and how to access it.

☐ **15.** Has discharge planning begun? Refer to Checklist 7.

DATE: _____6/12_____   **DAY # OF HOSPITALIZATION:** __2__

NURSES TODAY

Day Nurse: *Ann*   Shift Time: *7 AM-7 PM*

Night Nurse: *Donna*   Shift Time: *7 PM-7 AM*

Doctors seen today / Time: ☐

Medications on time and correct? ☐

Invasive devices (IV, catheter, ventilator, etc.) checked by nurse? ☑

Is there a removal date? ☐

What Happened Today? Refer to Daily Reminders Checklist.

Saw Dr. Harder at 3 P.M. He increased pain meds—

changed to morphine drip.

Had x-ray of shoulder/jaw at noon—requested copies.

Met Patty Smith—patient advocate. Helped us reach

orthopedic surgeon to discuss surgery.

Food all wrong. Soft diet for jaw but they keep

forgetting.

RED FLAG

Lisa can't sleep. What can we do?

SAMPLE

DATE: _____   **DAY # OF HOSPITALIZATION:** _____

NURSES TODAY

Day Nurse: _____   Shift Time: _____

Night Nurse: _____   Shift Time: _____

Doctors seen today / Time: ☐

Medications on time and correct?   ☐

Invasive devices (IV, catheter, ventilator, etc.) checked by nurse? ☐

Is there a removal date?   ☐

What Happened Today? Refer to Daily Reminders Checklist.

_____

_____

_____

_____

_____

_____

_____

_____

_____

RED FLAG

DATE: _____   **DAY # OF HOSPITALIZATION:** _____

NURSES TODAY

Day Nurse: _____   Shift Time: _____

Night Nurse: _____   Shift Time: _____

Doctors seen today / Time: ☐

Medications on time and correct? ☐

Invasive devices (IV, catheter, ventilator, etc.) checked by nurse? ☐

Is there a removal date? ☐

What Happened Today? Refer to Daily Reminders Checklist.

_____

_____

_____

_____

_____

_____

_____

_____

RED FLAG

DATE: _____   **DAY # OF HOSPITALIZATION:** _____

NURSES TODAY
_____

Day Nurse: _____   Shift Time: _____

Night Nurse: _____   Shift Time: _____

Doctors seen today / Time: □

Medications on time and correct? □

Invasive devices (IV, catheter, ventilator, etc.) checked by nurse? □

Is there a removal date? □

What Happened Today? Refer to Daily Reminders Checklist.

_____

_____

_____

_____

_____

_____

_____

_____

RED FLAG

DATE: _____   **DAY # OF HOSPITALIZATION:** _____

NURSES TODAY

Day Nurse: _____   Shift Time: _____

Night Nurse: _____   Shift Time: _____

Doctors seen today / Time: ☐

Medications on time and correct? ☐

Invasive devices (IV, catheter, ventilator, etc.) checked by nurse? ☐

Is there a removal date? ☐

What Happened Today? Refer to Daily Reminders Checklist.

_____

_____

_____

_____

_____

_____

_____

_____

RED FLAG

DATE: _____ **DAY # OF HOSPITALIZATION:** _____

NURSES TODAY
_____

Day Nurse: _____ Shift Time: _____

Night Nurse: _____ Shift Time: _____

Doctors seen today / Time: ☐

Medications on time and correct? ☐

Invasive devices (IV, catheter, ventilator, etc.) checked by nurse? ☐

Is there a removal date? ☐

What Happened Today? Refer to Daily Reminders Checklist.

_____

_____

_____

_____

_____

_____

_____

_____

RED FLAG

DATE: _____   **DAY # OF HOSPITALIZATION:** _____

NURSES TODAY

Day Nurse: _____   Shift Time: _____

Night Nurse: _____   Shift Time: _____

Doctors seen today / Time: ☐

Medications on time and correct?   ☐

Invasive devices (IV, catheter, ventilator, etc.) checked by nurse? ☐

Is there a removal date?   ☐

What Happened Today? Refer to Daily Reminders Checklist.

_____

_____

_____

_____

_____

_____

_____

RED FLAG

DATE: _____   **DAY # OF HOSPITALIZATION:** ____

NURSES TODAY

Day Nurse: _____   Shift Time: _____

Night Nurse: _____   Shift Time: _____

Doctors seen today / Time: ☐

Medications on time and correct? ☐

Invasive devices (IV, catheter, ventilator, etc.) checked by nurse? ☐

Is there a removal date? ☐

What Happened Today? Refer to Daily Reminders Checklist.

_____

_____

_____

_____

_____

_____

_____

_____

RED FLAG

DATE: _____ **DAY # OF HOSPITALIZATION:** _____

NURSES TODAY
_____

Day Nurse: _____ Shift Time: _____

Night Nurse: _____ Shift Time: _____

Doctors seen today / Time: ☐

Medications on time and correct? ☐

Invasive devices (IV, catheter, ventilator, etc.) checked by nurse? ☐

Is there a removal date? ☐

What Happened Today? Refer to Daily Reminders Checklist.

_____

_____

_____

_____

_____

_____

_____

_____

RED FLAG

DATE: _____   **DAY # OF HOSPITALIZATION:** _____

NURSES TODAY

Day Nurse: _____   Shift Time: _____

Night Nurse: _____   Shift Time: _____

Doctors seen today / Time: ☐

Medications on time and correct?   ☐

Invasive devices (IV, catheter, ventilator, etc.) checked by nurse?   ☐

Is there a removal date?   ☐

What Happened Today? Refer to Daily Reminders Checklist.

_____

_____

_____

_____

_____

_____

_____

_____

RED FLAG

DATE: _____   **DAY # OF HOSPITALIZATION:** _____

NURSES TODAY

Day Nurse: _____   Shift Time: _____

Night Nurse: _____   Shift Time: _____

Doctors seen today / Time: ☐

Medications on time and correct?   ☐

Invasive devices (IV, catheter, ventilator, etc.) checked by nurse? ☐

Is there a removal date?   ☐

What Happened Today? Refer to Daily Reminders Checklist.

_____

_____

_____

_____

_____

_____

_____

_____

RED FLAG

DATE: _____ **DAY # OF HOSPITALIZATION:** _____

NURSES TODAY
_____

Day Nurse: _____ Shift Time: _____

Night Nurse: _____ Shift Time: _____

Doctors seen today / Time: ☐

Medications on time and correct? ☐

Invasive devices (IV, catheter, ventilator, etc.) checked by nurse? ☐

Is there a removal date? ☐

What Happened Today? Refer to Daily Reminders Checklist.

_____

_____

_____

_____

_____

_____

_____

_____

RED FLAG

DATE: _____   **DAY # OF HOSPITALIZATION:** _____

NURSES TODAY

Day Nurse: _____   Shift Time: _____

Night Nurse: _____   Shift Time: _____

Doctors seen today / Time: ☐

Medications on time and correct?   ☐

Invasive devices (IV, catheter, ventilator, etc.) checked by nurse? ☐

Is there a removal date?   ☐

What Happened Today? Refer to Daily Reminders Checklist.

_____

_____

_____

_____

_____

_____

_____

_____

RED FLAG

DATE: _____   **DAY # OF HOSPITALIZATION:** _____

NURSES TODAY

Day Nurse: _____   Shift Time: _____

Night Nurse: _____   Shift Time: _____

Doctors seen today / Time: ☐

Medications on time and correct?   ☐

Invasive devices (IV, catheter, ventilator, etc.) checked by nurse?   ☐

Is there a removal date?   ☐

What Happened Today? Refer to Daily Reminders Checklist.

_____

_____

_____

_____

_____

_____

_____

_____

RED FLAG

HOSPITAL SPOTLIGHT

A Spiritual Hand Can Help

My mother was heavily drugged with morphine after invasive surgery for pancreatic cancer. Morphine can change one's personality and in her case, my mom just got really mean—not her normal self at all. She especially turned her wrath on my father, her husband of forty years, who was at her bedside all day, every day. Her doctors didn't seem particularly disturbed by it but we were. My mom's church had always been central to her life, so I asked the minister whom she was closest to if she could visit my mom and try to help us all. Dad, a die-hard atheist, thought it was a pretty futile idea. But that minister was the only person who could comfort and quiet my mother over a few critical days. It was a true blessing for my family and, as the minister shared with me later, a blessing for her too.

Hospital Delirium Fact Sheet

The stats: most common complication among people ages 65 and over. Over 20 percent of **all** hospital patients. Up to 60 percent of those who have certain surgeries like hip replacements. Up to 80 percent of those treated in ICUs.

Signs: sudden change in mental status; difficulty focusing; impaired memory; restlessness; insomnia; daytime sleepiness; being too quiet.

Potential causes: drug interactions; undiagnosed urinary tract infections; dehydration; anemia; pneumonia; stress of illness or injury; disorienting hospital setting.

How family can help:

1. Ground the patient in familiar things—family photos, a favorite playlist, calm conversations about recent events in their life.
2. Use sensory aids—not using hearing aids, glasses, and dentures impacts a patient's ability to function.
3. Normalize day/night cycle and get moving, if possible. Ask for a bed by the window. Take your family member for a walk.
4. Promote hydration, nutrition, sleep—avoid sleeping pills, if possible.
5. Ask for a medication review. Certain meds, like sleeping pills or tranquilizers, that are commonly dispensed in hospitals can contribute to delirium. Is the patient's pain medication adequate?

ICU Family Information Fact Sheet

The Intensive Care Unit, or ICU, is the specialized hospital department that provides critical medical care to those patients with severe or life-threatening illness or injury. It can be an extremely intimidating place for both patients and families. That said, ICUs do make an effort to include family where and when they can. Below is a list of questions for family (and the patient, if conscious) to stay engaged with the ICU care team.

1. Do you and your family understand why you are in the ICU?
2. What is the diagnosis/prognosis? Diagnosis is identifying or giving a name to the disease or medical problem—why the move to ICU? Prognosis means estimating or predicting the outcome based on current treatment—in this case the goals for and duration of ICU care.
3. Who is on your ICU care team and what are their roles? Get contact information. Who is your day-to-day point person? Usually this is your nurse who generally has only two patients in the ICU.
4. When will the ICU care team give you regular updates? When do they round? Do they include family when rounding?
5. Let the ICU care team know who is the health-care proxy and family spokesperson. Give them your family contact information.
6. Confirm with the ICU team that they have any living wills or other advance care planning documents and that these are in the hospital chart.
7. Ask if the ICU care team can schedule regular family meetings to bring the family and care team together to review goals of care and answer questions.

8. Ask what the protocol is to prevent hospital delirium as up to 80 percent of all ICU patients can experience delirium because of the disorienting setting and intensive treatment protocol.

9. Keep track of all medications, medication schedules, and invasive medical devices.

10. Ask what family can and cannot do to help the care team: staying at bedside, talking to patient, hand-holding, reading stories, bringing in photos, gentle foot massages, playing music, and so on.

Discharge Plan

"*Medical science is focused on the here and now. The art of medicine, on the other hand, is always focused on the future because it is only the future that counts for the patient.*"

—Eric J. Cassell, *The Nature of Suffering*

Patients who reported they were not involved in their discharge planning and needs assessment had a 34 percent higher hospital readmission rate.

Patient Experience Journal 4, no. 2 (2017)

Failed handoffs during transitions in care are a long-standing, common problem in health care.

The Joint Commission, *Sentinel Event Alert* 58, September 12, 2017

☐ **1.** Find out as early as you can when you might be discharged and ask to meet with your discharge planner, most likely a social worker or case manager, as soon as possible. Your discharge planner works with your medical team to coordinate the care you need from the moment you leave the hospital with a focus on making your move from hospital to home or another facility safe.

☐ **2.** Know who is on your discharge team and what their roles are. Many people are involved with hospital discharge planning. Team members can include:

- **Your doctor/hospitalist** will be the one who signs off that you are medically ready for discharge. Your doctor will prescribe medications, order all rehab services—a transfer to a rehab facility or outpatient therapy, any skilled nursing, and home care services. Insurance will only pay for these services with a doctor's order because they are considered medically necessary.

- **Your nurse** will be your hands-on discharge team member to educate you about any medical tasks for wound care or invasive devices you may still need at discharge—surgical site, drains, ports, IVs, and so on. If you are going to need to learn a certain task, start watching how your nurse does it while you are in the hospital and ask questions now. Don't wait until the day of discharge. Your nurse will also go over all medications with you—make sure you understand!

- **Your social worker/case manager** is the point person on your discharge team—the discharge planner—who coordinates everything involved when you move from hospital to home or another facility. This can include outpatient follow-up services, skilled nursing care, home health care, and durable medical equipment for your home like a hospital bed, oxygen, or commode. The social worker contacts your insurance to see what is covered and will help with referrals and vendors if you need to pay out of pocket. They may also schedule follow-up doctor visits. You need to ask what your social worker will and won't put in place for you and what you need to do.

- **You and your family caregivers are very much a part of this discharge team.** A discharge to home requires involved family members as aftercare can be quite complex. Patients are now discharged sooner and sicker. Insurance at most pays for a limited amount of skilled nursing care and rarely for a home health aide. Your discharge team needs to understand and evaluate the full range of your aftercare needs; home environment, availability of family caregivers, etc.

- Add all contact info for the hospital discharge team, including home care agencies and equipment vendors, to Checklist 9. Modify the contact list where necessary but it is helpful to have all hospital-related contacts in one place.

☐ **3.** Have a family member present with you at *every* planning meeting and that you get clear written instructions at discharge. Leaving the hospital and the transition involved can be stressful. You need someone to listen with you, take notes, and speak up for you, if necessary, to ensure as much as possible that your needs and requests are guiding the decisions being made— whether you are being discharged to home (with or without some level of help) or a rehabilitation facility.

4. Discuss with both your doctor and nurses what you can generally expect the first few days and weeks after you are discharged home.

- When can you expect to resume your normal routine?
- How mobile will you be? Or should you be?
- Are sleep disturbances, night sweats, lack of appetite, or other physical symptoms normal for your situation in response to surgery, treatment, or anesthesia?
- Are feelings of anxiety, restlessness, depression—within reason—common emotional reactions in your doctor's experience, given what you might have gone through?
- What would be a red flag, abnormal event, or side effect that would be cause for alarm in your situation? Whom should you contact?

5. Review instructions with the discharge team for surgical care.

- Can you bathe? If so, how? Should you keep your wound from getting wet? What should you do in that case?
- Review and practice with your nurse and/or doctor your wound care instructions until you completely understand them.
- What physical symptoms are cause for concern and whom should you contact?
- What is the plan for removal of any stitches or staples, and has an appointment been made?

6. Review instructions for the proper care of any medical devices. You may be discharged tethered to IVs or with drains, ports, and the like, which need to be monitored closely for infection, leaks, or blockages, or you may be sent home in a cervical collar, body brace, sling, or cast.

- Remember any break in the skin barrier is susceptible to infection.
- Make sure you completely understand how to properly clean, change, and monitor devices that remain in you or attached to you. When can they be removed?
- What would be a red flag that something is wrong—such as an infection, leakage, or blockage? What are the possible symptoms? What should you do if something like that occurs?

7. **Make sure you really, really understand all instructions for medications that are to be continued at home. Review the hospital discharge medication list and schedule with your discharge team. Check and double-check the following:**
   - Have all changes in your medication been reviewed by you, your doctor, your nurse, and your family?
   - Should you resume any medications you were taking prehospitalization that might have been discontinued during your hospital stay?
   - Review all medication labels against written discharge instructions.
   - Make sure you understand the daily schedule, dosage, how to take (with food, etc.), side effects for all medications you will be taking.
   - Is there a special protocol for pain management? What should you do if you are home and you feel that your pain is getting away from you?
   - Make sure you are going home with your prescriptions filled. If not, make sure your physician has called in the order to your pharmacy and that your medication is in stock. Either have it delivered or have a family member pick it up *before* you are discharged.

- Now might be the time to consider a medication reminder app. See the Resources section in this book.
- Get a pill organizer and a pill cutter if necessary.
- See the Resources for medication charts to download.

8. **Plan with your social worker for all home care needs: follow-up medical appointments, outpatient rehabilitation, durable medical equipment, and home care services. Be clear on what follow-up care your social worker will coordinate and schedule, what the hospital will provide, and what you will need to do and when.**

- Has your doctor put in an order for a visiting nurse? How many visits per week? When is the first visit? For how many weeks (usually just two)? Who schedules appointments?
- Have you been approved for home care service? How many days/hours per week? When will it start/end? Who schedules visits?
- What equipment and supplies do you need at home— hospital bed, commode, oxygen, disposable gloves, shower chair, and the like? Who organizes this and pays for it?
- What outpatient physical therapy and/or other rehabilitation services will you need?
- Do you need to schedule follow-up doctor appointments?
- What about transportation home, to doctor visits, or therapy if needed?
- How long after discharge will the social worker coordinate home care services and issues for you (if at all)? Is this person your hospital contact for questions in follow-up care and, if so, for how long after discharge?
- If you don't have insurance coverage or need to pay out of pocket, can your social worker help you organize options and services before discharge?

☐ **9.** Make sure your primary care physician is brought into the loop before you leave the hospital and schedule a follow-up visit if they will be taking over care. Make sure all important reports, tests, and discharge summaries will be sent to your primary care physician. Will your social worker make this appointment or do you need to? Will the social worker arrange to send all medical records to your primary care physician?

☐ **10.** Will you have enough family support at home? Don't underestimate the amount of help you may need the first few days/weeks that you are home—from personal care to medication to accompanying you to doctor follow-ups or outpatient rehab.

☐ **11.** Get a list of referrals to help you if you need to organize more care after discharge to home: home health agencies, medical equipment vendors, community resources, meal services, transportation services. Your case worker/social worker may help you in organizing these services—ask them for help. You may have to pay for most, if not all, of these services out of pocket if your doctor has not prescribed them. That doesn't mean you won't need them.

☐ **12.** If you are being discharged to an acute rehabilitation hospital or skilled nursing facility, keep these items in mind:

- Your doctor needs to put in an order for inpatient rehab services if you need more intensive therapies and skilled nursing than can be provided at home.
- Rehab can include physical, occupational, and speech therapies.

- Insurance covers only a limited amount of time in rehab—usually a few weeks.
- Often patients who are older need to go to rehab to improve function *because* of the effects of a hospital stay: bed rest, hospital food, and sedative drugs take a toll.
- Rehab facilities will only take you if you meet their criteria—generally that you will improve with these intensive therapies.

13. Review carefully with your social worker/case manager what services and equipment needs will and will not be covered by your insurance.

14. Request all hospital medical and billing records now! It is much more difficult to get copies after you are discharged. You may not be able to access all records through the patient portal:
- Discharge summary and instructions
- An itemized hospital bill of charges to date
- Pathology reports
- All scans
- Surgical reports
- Progress notes
- Emergency room records

15. You can appeal your discharge if you think it is too soon and not safe. By law, the hospital needs to help you file this appeal with the appropriate entity and explain the process to you. See the Resources section.

Have a Rock-Solid Discharge Plan in Place Before You Leave the Hospital

My friend Robyn was sent home after having a hysterectomy for ovarian cancer with no prescription-strength pain medication. The resident handling her discharge told her husband that she should take ibuprofen as needed. She had two young children at home—a four-year-old and a three-month-old. By the time Robyn got home, she was in agony. Her husband called me in a panic. I rushed over to find Robyn curled up in a ball on her bed, almost unable to speak. I made her husband page her surgeon. There had been a mistake—a terrible one—with her discharge instructions: her pain medications had been omitted. Her surgeon immediately called in a rush prescription to her local pharmacy, but it took hours to get Robyn's pain under control and she suffered needlessly because of a serious medication error in her discharge instructions.

Notes

Discharge Plan

Insurance

"In our modern health-care industrial complex—and I am talking about the bureaucracies who try and herd you into the cheapest cattle car available, not the nurses and doctors who are on the frontlines— the emphasis is neither on health nor care, but the bottom line. It's our job, as patients, to resist with all our strength."

—Dana Jennings, "10 Lessons of Prostate Cancer," *New York Times,* "Well Blog," November 25, 2008

A new study from academic researchers found that 66.5 percent of all bankruptcies were tied to medical issues—either because of high costs or time out of work. An estimated 530,000 families turn to bankruptcy each year because of medical issues and bills, the research found.

"This Is the Real Reason Most Americans
File for Bankruptcy," CNBC.com,
February 11, 2019

1. Fill out the healthcare insurance information on page 119 immediately so that pertinent insurance ID card information and contact numbers for member services and hospital billing are handy for you and your family in a hard-copy format. Consider the following:

   - As in Checklist 1, task a family member with being your insurance and hospital billing point person.
   - Give them log-in information to your insurance and patient portal, if this makes sense based on your circumstances and needs.
   - Call both your insurance company and the hospital billing department and give them permission to speak to your family member on your behalf. This will allow your family member to address any issues (and there will be issues) that come up with billing, benefits, and claims in a timely fashion.
   - Pick someone who is extremely organized, trustworthy, and calm. Dealing with the costs of care requires a dogged determination mixed with utmost diplomacy.

2. Get in touch with your insurance company.
   - Always write down the date, time, name, and subject matter for every conversation you have with an insurance representative going forward. You can adapt the notes section here to use as a call log.
   - Make allies within your insurance company with anyone who is helpful—you will most likely need help navigating their system.

3. Ask your insurance company if you have been assigned a "case/care/utilization manager" or "health coach/advocate," someone who is typically assigned in the case of chronic illness or serious diagnosis.

They will be your go-to within the insurance company to confirm authorizations, help you understand benefits, expedite paperwork, file claims, and navigate denials or reimbursement disputes. Get in touch with them.

4. Be clear on the pre-certification approval process with your surgeon or specialist's office manager and confirm with your insurance company.
   - Make sure all providers (like radiologists and anesthesiologists) who might be involved with your care are in network.
   - Is the hospital in your insurance network? If the hospital is out of network, what percentage of the bill will the insurance company pay (80/20, 70/30, 50/50, for example)?

5. If your insurance is through your workplace, ask the benefits manager in your human resources (HR) department to help you understand and navigate your health benefit plan. Many companies are now working with independent patient-advocate services to help you with what is often the worst aspect of any hospital stay—the endless hassles from your insurance company. This can be an important resource.

6. Understand your financial obligations. What is your co-pay? (A co-pay applies to each medical service you receive.) What is your deductible? Do you have an out-of-pocket maximum? (This is the most you will have to pay.) Is there a lifetime maximum benefit? (This is the most the insurance company will pay.)

☐ **7.** Does your insurance company make payments based on UCR rates—usual, customary, and reasonable (which are insurance industry–dictated rates)—or actual hospital charges for your area? This amount can vary widely based on geographical location and can significantly impact what you must pay.

☐ **8.** Maintain Checklists 4–6. They serve as your record of all medications and medical treatment to match against every hospital bill. Check for clerical errors, discrepancies, double billing, and the like. As much as 80 percent of all hospital bills contain billing errors. Immediately alert the billing department of the hospital if there are any errors and begin their internal dispute process.

☐ **9.** Consider hiring an outside medical billing advocate to audit, negotiate, and resolve your medical bills. A professional advocate might be better equipped to navigate a byzantine system designed to be inscrutable. Generally, a professional patient advocate takes a percentage (usually 10 percent) of your overall reimbursement, which may well be worth it to you if the claims and denial process drags on.

☐ **10.** For the uninsured and underinsured:
- Remember *everything* is negotiable, including your hospital bill.
- Uninsured patients can be billed for a procedure up to three times more than the rate an insurance company has negotiated.
- Research the cost of your procedure at hospitals within your area. Fees can vary widely. See ClearHealthCosts

in the Resources section for comparison pricing of just about any procedure large or small.

- Ask for the best rate offered to insurance companies and set up a payment plan.
- Contact the hospital's Financial Assistance Office, if they have one.
- Enlist a patient advocacy organization whose mission is to help uninsured patients—see the Resources section. These organizations do not charge you and can advise you on accessible and affordable services, payment plans, and financial aid funds.
- Medical crowdfunding has become a common and often effective way to meet medical needs.

Insurance Information

Fill out the form on page 119 with your individual insurance details. This is a sample template—all member cards have different designations. Make a note of helpful contacts at your insurance company, your workplace (such as HR), and the hospital billing/financial assistance offices. You may need an ally to help you cut through red tape, get an approval, expedite a claim, and so on.

Primary Insurance Provider (adapt from your card info)

Name of policyholder:

DOB and SS# of policyholder*:

Member ID#:

Group#:

Claims phone number:

Contact:

Secondary Insurance Provider (adapt from your card info)

Name of policyholder:

DOB and SS# of policyholder*:

Member ID#:

Group#:

Claims phone number:

Contact:

Prescription Drug ID Card (adapt from your card info)

ID#:

RxGrp:

RxBin:

Employer human resources contact (name/phone/email for contact):

Hospital billing dept. contact (name/phone/email for contact):

*If you are not the policyholder—spouse, parent, etc.

Medical Billing Resources and Insurance Claims/Denials Resources

1. Patient Advocate Foundation (https://www.patientadvocate .org/): case managers provide one-on-one counseling on medical billing issues free of charge.

2. Hospital Cost Compare (https//www.hospitalcostcompare .com): website that compares what Medicare reimburses for procedures against what a hospital might charge you. Can be helpful in negotiating a better rate at your hospital.

3. Alliance of Claims Assistance Professionals (https://www .claims.org/refer.php): members provide medical claims assistance, patient advocacy, and uninsured cost of care negotiations.

4. ClearHealthCosts (https://clearhealthcosts.com): website with extensive price comparisons for just about any type of medical procedure—routine to acute care.

5. AdvoConnection Directory (https://advoconnection.com/): a source for locating professional health/patient advocates and care managers.

6. National Association of Healthcare Advocates (https:// www.nahac.com/find-an-advocate#!directory/map): another source for locating a health advocate.

Insurance Companies, Money, and Health

In 1993, my mother recuperated in the hospital for twenty-three days after complex and invasive surgery for pancreatic cancer. In 2007, my brother-in-law was discharged four days after complex and invasive open heart surgery.

After a serious bike accident in which she broke her jaw, six ribs, and her shoulder, Lisa C. got a bill from her insurance company for the $700 ambulance ride but they covered her surgery. It took her six months to get the claim paid.

Insurance

Notes

_____

_____

_____

_____

_____

_____

_____

_____

_____

_____

_____

_____

_____

_____

_____

Insurance

Doctor Contacts

Surgeons must be very careful
when they take the knife!
Underneath their fine incisions
Stirs the culprit...Life!

—Emily Dickinson

Researchers found that radiologists' reports were significantly more thorough in all cases when a photograph was attached to a patient's scan.

"Radiologist Adds a Human Touch: Photos," *New York Times*, April 6, 2009

How to adapt this contact list so that you will have all hospital-connected contacts in one place:

☐ **1.** Add all doctors and contact info—follow the prompts in the box.

☐ **2.** You may work very closely with some of the staff who report to them—residents, interns, and the like. They may be your point people for questions—find out.

☐ **3.** If your specialty doctors have their own nurse practitioner (NP) or physician's assistant (PA) on staff, this person is often your go-to for everyday questions with that specialist.

☐ **4.** Add your case manager/social worker to the hospital information page.

☐ **5.** Add your discharge information to the hospital information page.

HOSPITAL INFORMATION PAGE

Date of hospitalization: _____

MRN number: _____

Hospital name: _____

Address: _____

Main number: _____

Nurses' station number for your floor: _____

Nurse manager name and number
for your floor or unit: _____

Room number: _____

Room phone number: _____

Case manager: _____

Social worker: _____

Patient relations number (call if you have issues that
are not being addressed): _____

Rehab facility if applicable: _____

Discharge instructions reviewed with: _____

Discharge services referrals (medical equipment, nursing
services, PT, etc.):

_____

_____

_____

_____

_____

Doctor name:

Specialty:

Typical time for rounds:

Office phone: Cell phone:

Email:

Office receptionist:

Nurse practitioner: NP contact info:

Physician's assistant: PA contact info:

Hospital resident/intern reporting to doctor:

Contact info:

Doctor name:

Specialty:

Typical time for rounds:

Office phone: Cell phone:

Email:

Office receptionist:

Nurse practitioner: NP contact info:

Physician's assistant: PA contact info:

Hospital resident/intern reporting to doctor:

Contact info:

Special notes:

Doctor Contacts

Doctor name: _____

Specialty: _____

Typical time for rounds: _____

Office phone: _____ Cell phone: _____

Email: _____

Office receptionist: _____

Nurse practitioner: _____ NP contact info: _____

Physician's assistant: _____ PA contact info: _____

Hospital resident/intern reporting to doctor: _____

Contact info: _____

Doctor name: _____

Specialty: _____

Typical time for rounds: _____

Office phone: _____ Cell phone: _____

Email: _____

Office receptionist: _____

Nurse practitioner: _____ NP contact info: _____

Physician's assistant: _____ PA contact info: _____

Hospital resident/intern reporting to doctor: _____

Contact info: _____

Special notes: _____

_____

_____

Doctor name:

Specialty:

Typical time for rounds:

Office phone: Cell phone:

Email:

Office receptionist:

Nurse practitioner: NP contact info:

Physician's assistant: PA contact info:

Hospital resident/intern reporting to doctor:

Contact info:

Doctor name:

Specialty:

Typical time for rounds:

Office phone: Cell phone:

Email:

Office receptionist:

Nurse practitioner: NP contact info:

Physician's assistant: PA contact info:

Hospital resident/intern reporting to doctor:

Contact info:

Special notes:

Doctor name: _____

Specialty: _____

Typical time for rounds: _____

Office phone: _____ Cell phone: _____

Email: _____

Office receptionist: _____

Nurse practitioner: _____ NP contact info: _____

Physician's assistant: _____ PA contact info: _____

Hospital resident/intern reporting to doctor: _____

Contact info: _____

Doctor name: _____

Specialty: _____

Typical time for rounds: _____

Office phone: _____ Cell phone: _____

Email: _____

Office receptionist: _____

Nurse practitioner: _____ NP contact info: _____

Physician's assistant: _____ PA contact info: _____

Hospital resident/intern reporting to doctor: _____

Contact info: _____

Special notes: _____

_____

_____

Doctor name:

Specialty:

Typical time for rounds:

Office phone: Cell phone:

Email:

Office receptionist:

Nurse practitioner: NP contact info:

Physician's assistant: PA contact info:

Hospital resident/intern reporting to doctor:

Contact info:

Doctor name:

Specialty:

Typical time for rounds:

Office phone: Cell phone:

Email:

Office receptionist:

Nurse practitioner: NP contact info:

Physician's assistant: PA contact info:

Hospital resident/intern reporting to doctor:

Contact info:

Special notes:

Doctor name:

Specialty:

Typical time for rounds:

Office phone: Cell phone:

Email:

Office receptionist:

Nurse practitioner: NP contact info:

Physician's assistant: PA contact info:

Hospital resident/intern reporting to doctor:

Contact info:

Doctor name:

Specialty:

Typical time for rounds:

Office phone: Cell phone:

Email:

Office receptionist:

Nurse practitioner: NP contact info:

Physician's assistant: PA contact info:

Hospital resident/intern reporting to doctor:

Contact info:

Special notes:

The Connection Between Doctor and Patient

Dory F. was diagnosed with stage 4 liver cancer. Miraculously, she pulled through complex invasive surgery and is doing well today. When I met with her while I was working as a patient advocate in her hospital, she told me the single most important thing that kept her spirits up during her hospital stay was her daily email exchange with her chief surgeon—just a line or two shared between the two of them created a deep and healing connection for her.

Family & Friends Contacts

"Have the courage to use your own understanding."

—Immanuel Kant

A 2015 American Society for Quality survey found that 83 percent of patients desired improved communications between patients and hospital caregivers as a priority for improved patient experience.

Some things to consider as you fill out your Family & Friends Contacts list:

☐ **1.** Which family members will be your primary advocates at bedside while you are in the hospital?

☐ **2.** Who is your health-care proxy?

☐ **3.** Who is the family spokesperson?

☐ **4.** Who can help you with insurance and billing questions?

☐ **5.** Who can help you on the home front?

Name: _____

Cell: _____ Landline: _____

Email: _____

Special notes: _____

_____

Name: _____

Cell: _____ Landline: _____

Email: _____

Special notes: _____

_____

Name: _____

Cell: _____ Landline: _____

Email: _____

Special notes: _____

_____

Name: _____

Cell: _____ Landline: _____

Email: _____

Special notes: _____

_____

Name:

Cell: _____ Landline: _____

Email: _____

Special notes: _____

_____

Name:

Cell: _____ Landline: _____

Email: _____

Special notes: _____

_____

Name:

Cell: _____ Landline: _____

Email: _____

Special notes: _____

_____

Name:

Cell: _____ Landline: _____

Email: _____

Special notes: _____

_____

Name:

Cell: _____ Landline: _____

Email: _____

Special notes: _____

_____

Name:

Cell: _____ Landline: _____

Email: _____

Special notes: _____

_____

Name:

Cell: _____ Landline: _____

Email: _____

Special notes: _____

_____

Name:

Cell: _____ Landline: _____

Email: _____

Special notes: _____

_____

Family & Friends Contacts

Name:

Cell: _____ Landline: _____

Email: _____

Special notes: _____

_____

Name:

Cell: _____ Landline: _____

Email: _____

Special notes: _____

_____

Name:

Cell: _____ Landline: _____

Email: _____

Special notes: _____

_____

Name:

Cell: _____ Landline: _____

Email: _____

Special notes: _____

_____

Name:

Cell: Landline:

Email:

Special notes:

Name:

Cell: Landline:

Email:

Special notes:

Name:

Cell: Landline:

Email:

Special notes:

Name:

Cell: Landline:

Email:

Special notes:

PRN = Patient Receives Nothing

My husband, David, broke his neck and back in a terrible bicycle accident last week, so I know firsthand the worry, fear, frustration, and stress of trying to participate in the hospital care of a family member who has suffered a traumatic injury during a pandemic when communication is severely limited. We all understand the strict no-visitor policies across the nation's and the world's hospitals, but my experience underscores how essential it is for families to be actively engaged in their loved one's care and hospitals need to find a work-around.

In patient advocacy circles we ruefully describe the medicine abbreviation PRN as "patient receives nothing." In medical jargon, PRN means "as needed." In the real world of the hospital, this prescription directive is most often the order for pain medicine; in other words, the patient recovering from open heart surgery or a broken back, or anything else for that matter, needs to have the wherewithal to *ask* for pain medication. When my husband first arrived at the emergency room in a neck and back brace he was put on a morphine drip. Ten hours later, when he was moved to the surgical unit, the morphine was stopped and pain medicine "as needed" was instituted. Yet, no one made that clear to my husband (who, mind you, was concussed and immobilized). As a result, over the course of the next twenty long hours he received *no* pain medication—none. My husband assumed that the muscle relaxant he was given every four hours was actually his pain medication and that he would have to make do.

I had been calling the hospital regularly, attempting to connect with any member of his health-care team. David finally reached me at 6 a.m. in tears because of his pain. I told him to call for his nurse and put me on speaker phone. His lovely nurse was horrified that this failure of communication had caused extreme and completely avoidable suffering for my husband. Had I been at his bedside, I would have reviewed all his medications and care goals with his doctors and nurses as they rounded. I would have been able to manage and monitor his care and actively partner with his care team. Workarounds to involve families remotely in the care of their loved ones are essential to protect the safety and promote the comfort of patients—who are always people first, patients second.

Resources

Books About Illness and Healing, the Doctor/Patient Relationship, and Caregiving

Broyard, Anatole. *Intoxicated by My Illness*. New York: Ballantine Books, 1992.

Butler, Katy. *Knocking on Heaven's Door*. New York: Scribner, 2013.

Butler, Katy. *The Art of Dying Well*. New York: Scribner, 2019.

Cassell, Eric J. *The Nature of Suffering and the Goals of Medicine*. New York: Oxford University Press, 2004.

Epstein, Ronald. *Attending: Medicine, Mindfulness, and Humanity*. New York: Scribner, 2017.

Gawande, Atul. *Being Mortal: Medicine and What Matters in the End*. New York: Picador, 2014.

Gawande, Atul. *Better: A Surgeon's Notes on Performance*. New York: Picador, 2009.

Gillick, Muriel R. *The Caregiver's Encyclopedia: A Compassionate Guide to Caring for Older Adults*. Baltimore: Johns Hopkins University Press, 2020.

Groopman, Jerome. *The Anatomy of Hope: How People Prevail in the Face of Illness*. New York: Random House, 2004.

Nuland, Sherwin B. *How We Die: Reflections on Life's Final Chapter*. New York: Vintage, 1993.

Ofri, Danielle. *What Patients Say, What Doctors Hear*. Boston: Beacon Press, 2017.

The Importance of Checklists

Gawande, Atul. *The Checklist Manifesto: How to Get Things Right*. New York: Picador, 2011.

Pronovost, Peter and Eric Vohr. *Safe Patients, Smart Hospitals: How One Doctor's Checklist Can Help Us Change Health Care from the Inside Out*. New York: Hudson Street Press, 2010.

Important Government Health-Related Websites

Centers for Disease Control and Prevention (https://www.cdc.gov/)

Centers for Medicare and Medicaid Services (https://www.cms.gov/)

HealthCare.gov (https://www.healthcare.gov/): insurance exchange to shop for and enroll in affordable insurance plans

Health.gov (https://health.gov/): portal for health-related resources and news from the U.S. government

Medicare.gov (https://www.medicare.gov/): official U.S. government site for all manner of information on plans, coverage, benefits, claims, appeals

National Center for Complementary and Integrative Medicine (https://www.nccih.nih.gov/): sizeable website of vetted information under the auspices of the National Institutes of Health

National Institutes of Health (https://www.nih.gov/): extensive health information, lists of clinical trials, and chronic disease and cancer registries

Help for Patient/Consumer

Choosing Wisely (https://www.choosingwisely.org/): organization whose mission is to promote conversations between clinicians and patients by helping patients choose treatments that are evidence-based, necessary, and free from harm

Medicare Rights Center (https://www.medicarerights.org/): national, nonprofit consumer service organization whose mission is to ensure access to affordable health care for older adults and people with disabilities; largest independent source for rights and benefits and help navigating the Medicare system

State Health Insurance Assistance Program (https://www.shiptacenter.org/): helps people navigate Medicare with state-specific guidance

Medical Billing Resources and Insurance Claims/ Denials Resources (from Checklist 8)

Patient Advocate Foundation (https://www.patientadvocate.org/): case managers provide one-on-one counseling on medical billing issues free of charge

Hospital Cost Compare (https//www.hospitalcostcompare.com): website that compares what Medicare reimburses for procedures against what a hospital might charge you; can be helpful in negotiating a better rate at your hospital

Alliance of Claims Assistance Professionals (https://www.claims.org /refer.php): members provide medical claims assistance, patient advocacy, and uninsured cost of care negotiations

Comparison Shopping and Price Transparency

ClearHealthCosts (https://clearhealthcosts.com): extensive price comparisons for just about any type of medical procedure that can be helpful in finding hospitals and negotiating a bill

National Directories for Patient Advocates

Hiring a private advocate to help you and your family navigate complex care may be helpful.

Verywell Health (https://www.verywellhealth.com/how-to-find-and -choose-a-patient-or-health-advocate-2614923): article about finding and interviewing a patient advocate

AdvoConnection Directory (https://advoconnection.com/): national directory of patient advocates

National Association of Healthcare Advocates (https://www.nahac .com/find-an-advocate#!directory/map): national directory

Advance Care Planning, Living Wills, and Health-Care Proxy Information

American Bar Association, Tool Kit for Health Care Advance Planning (https://ambar.org/agingtoolkit): free tool kit with information on how to choose a health-care proxy, a conversation script, and other useful tips and resources

MedicareInteractive.org (https://www.medicareinteractive.org/get-answers /planning-for-medicare-and-securing-quality-care/preparing-for -future-health-care-needs/health-care-proxies): powered by Medicare Rights Center—an easy-to-use website loaded with useful information

Caring Info (https://www.nhpco.org/patients-and-caregivers/table): a program sponsored by the National Hospice and Palliative Care Organization that provides state-specific forms

Five Wishes (https://fivewishes.org/): accessible, easy-to-understand information on advance care planning

AARP (https://www.aarp.org/caregiving/financial-legal/free-printable -advance-directives/): free advance directives by state and detailed guidance

The Conversation Project (https://theconversationproject.org/): easy-to- understand and -navigate website dedicated to helping family and friends talk about choices for medical care and end-of-life planning

National POLST (https://polst.org): interactive website that provides detailed state-by-state requirements and regulations on portable medical orders—commonly known as POLST (Physician Orders for Life-Sustaining Treatment) or MOLST (Medical Orders for Life-Sustaining Treatment) forms—that document specific choices for medical interventions, signed by your physician or a physician in a hospital and added to your medical chart

Palliative Care Information

Get Palliative Care (https://getpalliativecare.org/): consumer-oriented website for patients living with serious illness and their families that provides clear and comprehensive information and resources for this specialized medical care focusing on symptom manage- ment and quality of life

Choosing Wisely (https://www.choosingwisely.org/wp-content/uploads /2018/02/Palliative-Care-AAHPM.pdf): the organization's resource page on palliative care

Useful Hospital Website

Mayo Clinic (https://www.mayoclinic.org/): comprehensive informa- tion on just about any health issue

Medication Apps and Downloadable Lists: Tracking, Reminders, and Side Effects

Medisafe (https://www.medisafeapp.com/): medication reminder app

CareZone (https://carezone.com/home): enables you to scan your pill bottles for an instant medication list that you can share with doctors and family

AARP (https://www.aarp.org/health/drugs-supplements/info-2007/my _personal_medication_record.html): a downloadable medication list

Notes

Introduction Statistics Sources

More than 36 million Americans are admitted to the hospital each year.

Fast Facts on US Hospitals, 2020, American Hospital Association: https://www.aha.org/statistics/fast-facts-us-hospitals

A hospital patient, on average, is subject to one medication error per day.

Patient and Safety Quality: An Evidence-Based Handbook for Nurses, "Medication Reconciliation": https://www.ncbi.nlm.nih.gov/books/NBK2648/

Every six minutes a patient dies in an American hospital from a hospital-acquired infection—an infection acquired after admission.

Hospital Acquired Infections, americansmadandangry.org

Index

AARP Bulletin Today, 36
acupuncture, 42
advance directive
    at hospital admission, 29
    in ICU family information fact sheet,
        98
adverse patient events, harm or death
        from, 4
AdvoConnection Directory, 120
aide/patient ratio, 37
The Aiken Study, 36
air-conditioning, in hospitals, 30
allergies, to medications, 19
Alliance of Claims Assistance
        Professionals, 120
American Academy of Sleep Medicine,
        46
Anatomy of an Illness (Cousins), xi
anemia, hospital delirium from, 97
anesthesia
    discharge plan and, 105
    side effects of, 21
Annas, George J., 11
antibacterial wipes, in hospital room,
        39
antipsychotics, xxi, xxv, xxvi
anxiety, discharge plan and, 105
appeal, of discharge, 109
appetite, discharge plan and, 105
apps
    for family meetings, 18, 31
    for medications, 19

bankruptcies, 114
bathing
    in discharge plan, 105
    hospital aides for, 37
bed
    discharge plan and, 104, 107
    hospital delirium and, 97
    in hospital room, 38
    pressure sores from, 80
bed rest
    in hospital chaos, 32
    rehabilitation from, 109
bedside table, in hospital room, 38
blankets, in hospital room, 38
blood transfusions, 22
body brace, discharge plan and, 105
books
    by experts, xii
    at hospital admission, 29, 31
    in hospital room, 39
breathing tubes (machines)
    in daily journal, 80
    living will and, 15
    monitoring of, 5

call button, in hospital room, 38
CaringBridge.org, 18
case manager
    author's experience with, xxvi
    contact information for, 38
    discharge plan and, 41, 103–104, 109
    doctor contact information and, 125

case manager (*cont.*)
  for insurance, 109, 115–116
  patient portal and, 42
Cassell, Eric J., 101
casts, discharge plan and, 105
catheters
  in daily journal, 80
  hospital-acquired infections from,
    xxvii–xxviii
  monitoring of, 5
  surgical site management after, 21
cervical collar, discharge plan and, 105
The Checklist Manifesto (Gawande), 7
checklists
  of author, xxvi–xxvii
  communication in, 8
  for daily journal, 9, 77–96
  for daily medication log, 9, 61–75
  for discharge plan, 9, 21, 101–111
  for doctor contact information, 10,
    20–21, 123–133
  for family contact information, 10,
    135–144
  flowchart in, 8
  for friends contact information, 10,
    135–144
  for hospital admission, 8, 27–33
  for hospital stay, 8, 35–44
  for hospital-acquired infections,
    xxvii–xxviii
  for insurance, 9, 113–122
  for items to bring to hospital, 8, 27–33
  for master medication list, 9, 45–59
  for preparations before hospital admis-
    sion, 8, 11–25
  prompts in, 7–8
  summaries of, 8–10
  use of, 7–24
  user-friendliness of, 7
ClearHealthCosts, 120
climate control, in hospital room,
  38
comfort care, 6
  COVID-19 and, xiv
  in daily journal, 81
  by family, 37
  living will and, 16
  spiritual advisor visits for, 96
  by support system, 13
commode, discharge plan and, 104
communication
  breakdown of, 6

checklists for, 8
  by family spokesperson, 16–17
  on pain management, 50
  by support system, 13
  with whiteboard, 40–41
complementary care offerings, in hospi-
    tal stay, 42
constipation
  in daily journal, 80
  from hospital food, 41
contact information
  doctors, 10, 20–21, 37–38, 123–133
  family, 10, 98, 135–144
  friends, 10, 135–144
  at hospital admission, 29
  of hospital care team, 37–38, 98, 104
  for insurance, 115
  for nurses, 37–38
  for support system, 18
  on whiteboard, 40
contact tracing, xii
co-pay, with insurance, 116
Cousins, Norman, xi
COVID-19, xi, xiii–xiv
  isolation policies with, 17
CPR, living will and, 15
crosswords
  at hospital admission, 31
  in hospital room, 39
crowdfunding, 118

daily journal
  checklists for, 9, 77–96
  comfort care in, 81
  medication changes in, 79
  pain in, 79
  pain management in, 81
  surgery in, 79
daily medication log
  checklists for, 9, 61–75
  See also medication errors
daily reminders, 79–81
deaths
  from adverse patient events, 4
  from hospital-acquired infections, 4
  from medication errors, xvi
  from preventable diseases, 12
deductible, with insurance, 116
dehumanization, xxii
  as single greatest threat to patient's
    sanity, 6
dehydration, hospital delirium from, 97

demoralization, xxii
as single greatest threat to patient's sanity, 6
dentures
at hospital admission, 29
hospital delirium and, 97
in hospital room, 38
information to hospital care team on, 19
on whiteboard, 41
depression, discharge plan and, 105
diabetes
dietary restrictions for, xxi
insulin for, xx, xxi, xxiii
prednisone and, xv, xix
diagnosis
in ICU family information fact sheet, 98
insurance and, 115
physical examination for, 45
Dickinson, Emily, 123
dietary restrictions, for diabetes, xxi
discharge plan
appeal and, 109
bed and, 107
case manager and, 41, 103–104, 109
checklists for, 9, 21, 101–111
in daily journal, 81
doctors and, 103, 105
doctors contact information and, 125
family and, 104, 108
home health care and, 9, 103, 104, 107
hospital care team contact information and, 104
hospitalists and, 103
insurance and, 104, 107
invasive medical devices in, 103
medical records and, 109
medications in, 106–107
nurses and, 103, 105
pain management in, 106, 110
patient portal and, 109
preparations for, 41–42
primary care physician and, 108
readmissions after, 102
referrals and, 108
rehabilitation and, 9, 103, 104, 108–109
skilled nursing care, 103–104, 108–109
social workers and, 41, 103–104, 107, 109
for surgery, 105

doctor-patient relationship, 133
doctors
discharge plan and, 103, 105
as hospitalists, 37
medication review with, 47
thanks to, 42
visits by, 36
doctors contact information, 37–38
case manager and, 125
checklists for, 10, 20–21, 123–133
discharge plan and, 125
social workers and, 125
doctors rounds
in daily journal, 79
on whiteboard, 41
drains
discharge plan and, 103, 105
surgical site management after, 21
dressing, hospital aides for, 37

earbuds, in hospital room, 38
earplugs
at hospital admission, 30
in hospital room, 38
eBooks, at hospital admission, 29
electronic medical record (EMR), 22–23
endorphins, 43

family
blood transfusions and, 22
comfort care by, 6, 37
in daily journal, 81
discharge plan and, 104, 108
goals of care and, 14
at hospital admission, 29
in hospital room, 39
in hospital stay, 42–43
living will and, 16
medication errors and, 75
patient portal and, 42
as support system, 13
family contact information
checklists for, 10, 135–144
in ICU family information fact sheet, 98
family information fact sheet, for ICU, 80, 98–99
family meetings
apps for, 18, 31
with hospital care team, 81
in ICU family information fact sheet, 98

family spokesperson, 16–17
   in family contact information, 137
   in ICU family information fact sheet, 98
   insurance and, 115
   on whiteboard, 40
feeding, hospital aides for, 37
feeding tubes
   in daily journal, 80
   living will and, 15
finances, support system for, 18
flowchart, checklists for, 8
friends
   comfort issues and, 6
   contact information, 10, 135–144
   at hospital admission, 29
   in hospital stay, 42–43
   as support system, 13

games
   at hospital admission, 29, 31
   in hospital room, 39
Gawande, Atul, xxvii, 7
glasses
   at hospital admission, 29
   hospital delirium and, 97
   in hospital room, 38
   information to hospital care team on, 19
   on whiteboard, 41
goals of care, 13–14
Groopman, Jerome, 35

handoffs, 5
   in daily journal, 79
   failures in, 102
   support system at, 18
   on whiteboard, 40
hand-sanitizer
   at hospital admission, 30
   in hospital room, 38–39
handwashing, xiii–xiv
   by health-care providers, xxviii, 5
   in hospital room, 39–40
   hospital-acquired infections and, xxviii
headphones
   in hospital room, 38
   noise-cancelling, 32
health-care providers, 125
   handwashing by, xxviii, 5
   living will and, 15–16

   See also doctors; hospital care team; nurses; *specific providers*
health-care proxy, 14–15
   in family contact information, 137
   at hospital admission, 29
   in ICU family information fact sheet, 98
   on whiteboard, 40
Healthdesign.org, 28
hearing aids
   at hospital admission, 29
   hospital delirium and, 97
   in hospital room, 38
   information to hospital care team on, 19
   on whiteboard, 41
home health care, discharge plan and, 9, 103, 104, 107
hospital admissions
   checklists for, 8, 27–33
   family at, 29
   friends at, 29
   from medication errors, xvi, xxii
   patients' poor experience of, xx
   for preventable disease, 12
   previous experience with, 13–14
hospital aides
   aide/patient ratio for, 37
   thanks to, 42
hospital care team
   family meetings with, 81
   medication information to, 18–19
   thanks to, 42
   See also doctors; nurses
hospital care team contact information, 37–38
   discharge plan and, 104
   in ICU family information fact sheet, 98
Hospital Cost Compare, 120
hospital delirium
   in daily journal, 80
   fact sheet for, 97
   in ICU family information fact sheet, 99
hospital food, xxi, 37
   constipation from, 41
   rehabilitation from, 109
hospital information page, 126
hospital room
   cleanliness of, 39
   handwashing in, 39–40

practical considerations with, 38–39
whiteboard in, 40–41
hospital stay
checklists for, 8, 35–44
complementary care offerings in, 42
family in, 42–43
friends in, 42–43
hydration in, 41
nutrition in, 41
patient portal in, 42
spiritual advisor visits in, 42
touch in, 42, 43
hospital-acquired infections
checklists for, xxvii–xxviii
deaths from, 4
prevalence of, 28
hospitalists, 37
contact information for, 38
in daily journal, 79
discharge plan and, 103
hospitals
air-conditioning in, 30
chaos of, 32
noise levels in, 28
How Doctors Think (Groopman), 35
human error, as single greatest threat to
patient safety, 6
hydration
hospital delirium and, 97
in hospital stay, 41
hypnosis, 42

ICU. *See* Intensive Care Unit
infections
discharge plan and, 105, 106
from hospital rooms, 39
hospital-acquired, xxvii–xxviii, 4, 28
from invasive medical devices, 80
surgical site management after, 21
insulin, for diabetes, xx, xxi, xxiii
insurance
acute rehabilitation hospital and, 109
case manager for, 109, 115–116
checklists for, 9, 113–122
contact information for, 115
co-pay with, 116
deductible with, 116
discharge plan and, 104, 107
documented conversations with, 115
in family contact information, 137
family spokesperson and, 115
lifetime maximum benefit with, 116

Medicare, xxiii
pre-certification for, 116
resources for, 118–121
social workers and, 109
uninsured and underinsured, 117–118
usual, customary, and reasonable
(UCR) and, 117
through workplace, 116
insurance card, 29
Intensive Care Unit (ICU)
catheters in, xxviii
in daily journal, 80
family information fact sheet for, 80,
98–99
hospital delirium in, 78, 97
pain management in, 50
interpreters, on whiteboard, 41
invasive medical devices
in discharge plan, 103
in ICU family information fact sheet,
99
infections from, 80
isolation policies, with COVID-19, 17
items to bring to hospital, checklists, 8,
27–33
IV
in daily journal, 80
discharge plan and, 103, 105
monitoring of, 5
surgical site management after, 21

*JBI Database of Systematic Reviews and
Implementation*, 12
Jennings, Dana, 113
jewelry, at hospital admission, 31
The Joint Commission, 102
*Journal of Community Hospital Internal
Medicine Perspectives*, 46
Journal of Patient Safety, 12
*Journal of the American Medical Associa-
tion*, 36

key moments, support system for, 18

laughter, 42–43
lifetime maximum benefit, with insurance, 116
light-touch massage, 42
living will, 15–16
in ICU family information fact sheet,
98

massage, 42
master medication list
  checklists for, 9, 45–59
  filling out guide for, 48–49
medical billing
  bankruptcies from, 114
  errors in, 117
  resources for, 118–121
medical decision maker, 14–15
  as family spokesperson, 17
medical implants, information to hospital care team on, 19
medical records
  discharge plan and, 109
  EMR, 22–23
  health-care proxy and, 15
Medicare, uncovered care by, xxiii
medication errors
  deaths from, xvi
  from distraction, 62
  family and, 75
  hospital admissions from, xvi, xxii
  from lack of monitoring, xxi
  on night shift, 62
  per day, 4
  with prednisone, xv–xviii
  prevalence of, 46
medication side effects, 21, 48, 49
  discharge plan and, 106
medications, xv–xviii, xix, xxiii, 96
  abbreviations for, 49
  allergies to, 19
  apps for, 19
  changes to, 47
in daily journal, 79
  daily medication log, 9, 61–75
  discharge plan and, 103, 106–107
  hospital delirium and, 97
  in ICU family information fact sheet, 99
  information to hospital care team, 18–19
  master medication list, 9, 45–59
  for pain management, 22
  pill organizers and splitters for, 107
  polypharmacy and, 47–48
  review of, 47
  safety rights for, 63
  special instructions for, 49
  start and end dates for, 49
  See also pain management
morphine, 96

My Import Health Information, 24
  at hospital admission, 29
  for support system, 18

National Association of Healthcare
    Advocates, 120
National Center for Biotechnology Information, 62
The Nature of Suffering (Cassell), 101
night shift
  in daily journal, 79
  medication errors on, 62
night sweats, discharge plan and, 105
noise levels, in hospitals, 28
noise-cancelling headphones, at hospital
    admission, 32
NP. See nurse practitioner
Nuland, Sherwin, 45
nurse practitioner (NP), 125
nurse/patient ratio, 37
nurses
contact information for, 37–38
  in daily journal, 79
  discharge plan and, 103, 105
  for home health care, 107
  inadequate staffing of, 36
  medication review with, 47
  patient portal and, 42
  rounds of, on whiteboard, 40
  skilled nursing care, 103–104, 108
  thanks to, 42
nutrition, 37
  dietary restrictions, for diabetes, xxi
  hospital delirium and, 97
  in hospital stay, 41
  . See hospital food

occupational therapy
  in daily journal, 79
  discharge plan and, 108
On Being Ill (Woolf), 77
Osler, William, 61
oxygen, discharge plan and, 104, 107

PA. See physician's assistant
pain
  in daily journal, 79, 80
  sleep and, 46
pain management
  communication on, 50
  in daily journal, 81
  in discharge plan, 106, 110

PRN for, 143–144
  after surgery, 22
pajamas, at hospital admission, 30
palliative care. *See* comfort care
Patient Advocate Foundation, 120
Patient Experience Journal, 102
patient portal
  discharge plan and, 109
  in hospital stay, 42
patient receives nothing (PRN), 143–144
Patient Safety Week, xiii
patient-centered care, xii–xiii
payment plans, 118
pet therapy, 42
phone (hospital's), 38
phone (with charger)
  at hospital admission, 29
  in hospital room, 38
  safety of, 31
photo ID, 29
photographs
  at hospital admission, 31
  hospital delirium and, 97
  radiologists and, 124
physical examination, for diagnosis, 45
physical therapy
  in daily journal, 79
  discharge plan and, 108
physician's assistant (PA), 125
pill cutters, 107
pill organizers, 107
playlists
  at hospital admission, 29
  hospital delirium and, 97
  in hospital room, 39
pneumonia, hospital delirium from, 97
podcasts, at hospital admission, 29
polypharmacy, 47–48
ports
  in daily journal, 80
  discharge plan and, 105
  surgical site management after, 21
PPE, xii
pre-certification, for insurance, 116
prednisone
  medication errors with, xv–xviii
  psychosis from, xix, xxiii
pressure sores, in daily journal, 80
preventable disease, hospital admissions
    for, 12
primary care physician, discharge plan
    and, 108

PRN. *See* patient receives nothing
probiotics, 41
prognosis, in ICU family information
    fact sheet, 98
prompts, checklists for, 7–8
Pronovost, Peter, xxvii–xxviii
protected health information, patient
    portal and, 42
psychiatric ward, xxiv–xvi
psychosis, from prednisone, xix, xxiii

radiologists, photographs and, 124
reading glasses, at hospital admission, 29
referrals, discharge plan and, 108
rehabilitation
  discharge plan and, 9, 103, 104, 107,
      108–109
  social workers and, 107
Reiki, 42
restlessness
  discharge plan and, 105
  hospital delirium and, 97
resuscitation, living will and, 15
The Rights of Patients (Annas), 11
robe, at hospital admission, 30

Sentinel Event Alert, 102
shower chair, discharge plan and, 107
skilled nursing care, discharge plan and,
    103–104, 108
sleep
  discharge plan and, 105
  hospital delirium and, 97
  pain and, 46
sleep mask
  at hospital admission, 30, 32
  in hospital room, 38
slings, discharge plan and, 105
social workers
  author's experience with, xxvi
  contact information for, 38
  discharge plan and, 41, 103–104, 107,
      109
  doctor contact information and, 125
  insurance and, 109
  rehabilitation and, 107
socks, at hospital admission, 30
The Soul of Medicine (Nuland), 45
speech therapy, discharge plan and, 108
spiritual advisor visits
  for comfort care, 96
  in hospital stay, 42

spokesperson. *See* family spokesperson
stress of illness or injury, hospital delir-
    ium from, 97
Sudoku
    at hospital admission, 31
    in hospital room, 39
support system, 13
    organization of, 17–18
    after surgery, 22, 23
    See also family; friends
surgery
    annual number of, 4
    in daily journal, 79
    details of, 20
    discharge plan for, 105
    outcome of, 21
    pain management after, 22
    scheduling of, 19–20
    side effects of, 21
    site management after, 21
    support system after, 22, 23
surgical sites
    in daily journal, 80
    discharge plan and, 103, 105, 106

tablet or laptop computer (and charger),
    at hospital admission, 31, 32
temporal arteritis, xiv–xv
"10 Lessons of Prostate Cancer"
    (Jennings), 113

thanks, to hospital care team, 42
toileting, hospital aides for, 37
toiletries, at hospital admission,
    30–31
touch, in hospital stay, 42, 43
transportation, discharge plan and,
    107
treatment plans, changes to, 5
TV, in hospital room, 38

UCR. *See* usual, customary, and
    reasonable
underinsured, 117–118
uninsured, 117–118
urinary tract infections, hospital
    delirium from, 97
user-friendliness, of checklists, 7
usual, customary, and reasonable (UCR),
    insurance and, 117

ventilators, in daily journal, 80
visits
    by doctors, 36
    by spiritual advisors, 42, 96
    staggering of, 18

wallet, at hospital admission, 31
whiteboard, in hospital room, 40–41
Woolf, Virginia, 77
workplace, insurance through, 116

About the Author

A former producer, director, and vice president of music video production for several major record labels, Elizabeth Bailey holds a master of health advocacy from Sarah Lawrence College. She worked as a patient advocate at a major teaching hospital and now consults privately. She lives in New York City with her husband and son.